LEGENDS

CLARK GABLE

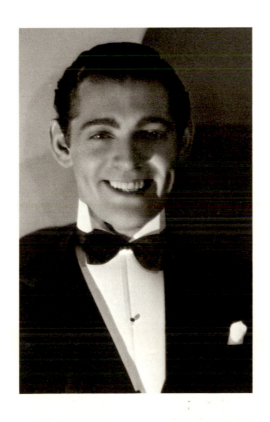

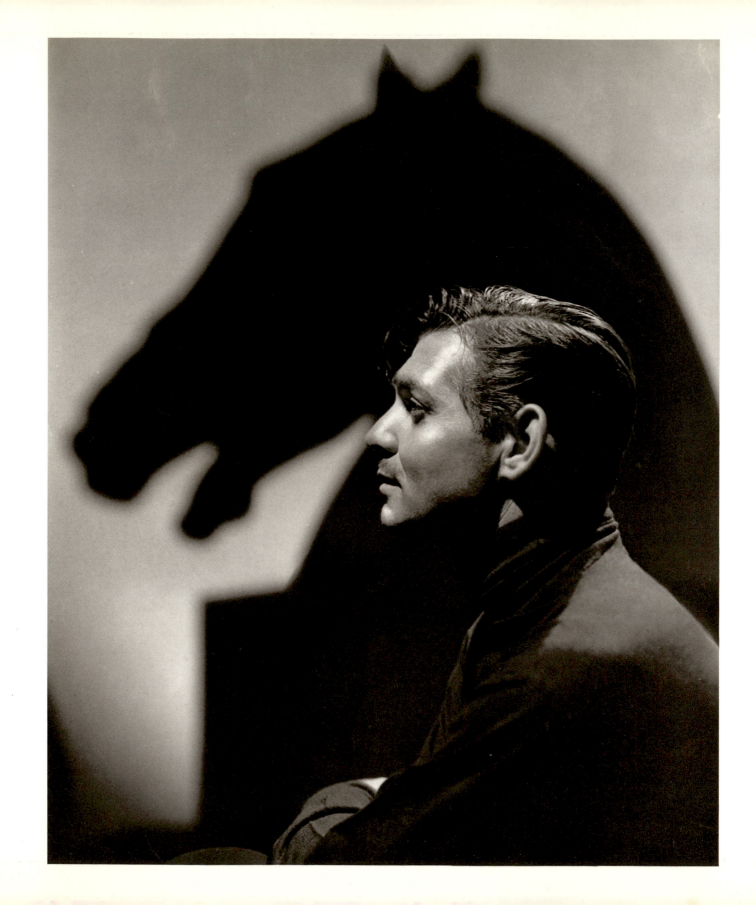

CLARK GABLE

INTRODUCTION BY
JAMES CARD
SERIES EDITOR
JOHN KOBAL

Photographs from
THE KOBAL COLLECTION

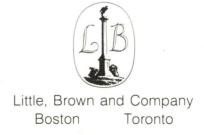

Little, Brown and Company
Boston   Toronto

To Joan Crawford whose presence
has illuminated so many movies
with and without Clark Gable
                              J.K.

I would like to thank Ben Carbonetto; Mark Ricci,
Memory Shop; Mary Corliss, Museum of Modern Art; Mark Viera;
and Brian Rule, C.I.S. for their contributions to this book.
                                          John Kobal

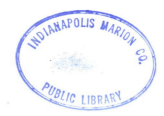

Library of Congress Catalog Card No. 85–82203

First American Edition

Designed by Craig Dodd

Printed in Italy

CONTENTS

 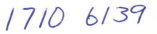

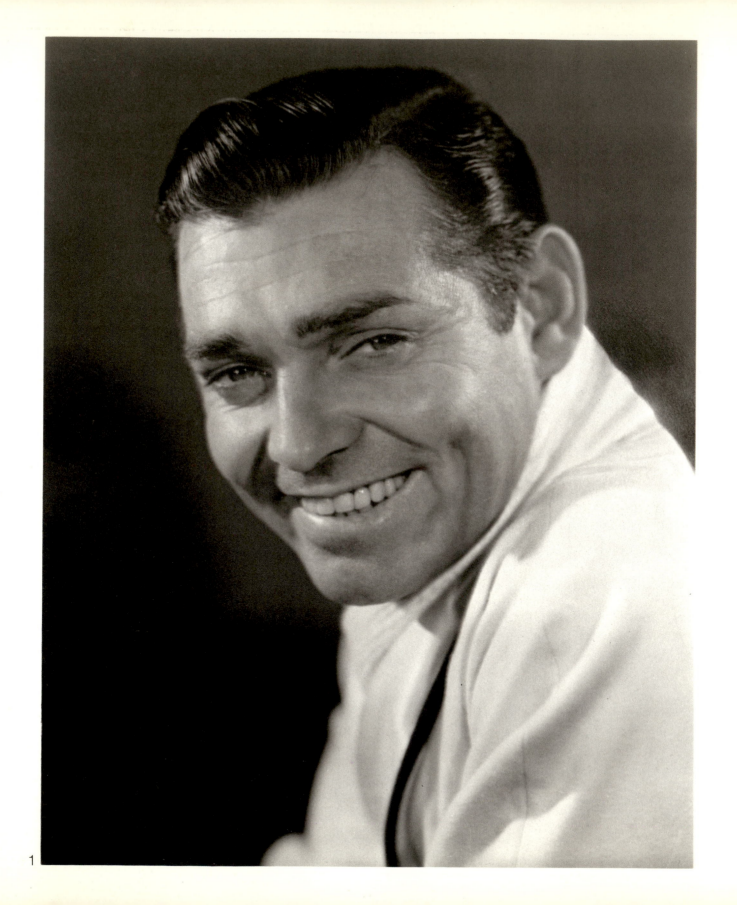

1

CLARK GABLE

There are elusive mysteries about the career of Clark Gable. There are questions that have driven each of his biographers to more speculation than should be expected in describing the life of one of filmdom's most visible and seemingly uncomplicated celebrities.

His very beginning cannot be determined with provable certainty. In both Meadville Pennsylvania and Cadiz Ohio there are official certifications of the birth of Clark Gable on the first day of February, 1901. But if there is documentary doubt about his birthplace, no uncertainty troubles today's citizens of grimy, economically blighted Cadiz whose inhabitants mis-pronounce the name of their town, calling it 'Catas' – as in 'catastrophic'.

On 1 February 1986, some two hundred assembled in unpleasant weather, late in the afternoon, to attend ceremonies dedicating a monument to Clark Gable on the site of a razed building where, according to Cadiz lore, Clark Gable was born to Adeline Hershelman Gable, a frail amateur artist who only nine months after the birth of her only child, died at the age of thirty-one.

The unveiling of the monument to Clark Gable was, of course, accompanied by the inevitable proclamations by local politicians. The chairman of the event read a fine letter from President Ronald Reagan, praising Clark Gable for having volunteered for active duty during the Second World War even though he had been well past the age when hazardous action would have been expected of him. Then there was a United States congressman, a Douglas Applegate who looked amazingly like a young Richard Nixon. Congressman Applegate managed to harangue the restless and shivering crowd with misinformation about the career of the honoree that was remarkable, even for a politician. For some reason, he went out of his way to insist that Gable had never appeared in silent films. (He had been in at least four.)

Saddest aspect of the event was the frequently expressed opinion that establishing the Gable monument in Cadiz would bring tourists streaming to that dismal spot, expending voyagers' dollars in amounts sufficient to help ease the woes of a community that once existed by mining coal – now no longer a much wanted fuel. Cadiz boasts of only one other celebrated son – General George Custer. By the looks of the General Custer Hotel in Cadiz, the fame of the ill-fated Indian fighter has brought no substantial group of his admirers to Cadiz since the Battle of Little Big Horn.

A far more appropriate location for a Gable monument would have been eight miles away in Hopedale Ohio where, from his mother's death until he was sixteen, Clark Gable spent the formative years of his boyhood. It seems incredible that there could be a town more dreary than Cadiz, but Hopedale is hopelessly so. Clinging to steep, eroded hillsides, even today the streets of Hopedale are muddy and unpaved. But the Gable home, built by Clark's father William in 1905, still stands solidly and rather handsomely, one of the three or four dwellings in all Hopedale that are not crumbling, ready to slide down the hillside slopes in desperate disrepair.

A visit to Hopedale gives one a clue as to why Clark Gable, at the very peak of his fabulous career, would describe himself to an interviewer as 'just a lucky slob from Ohio'. Even as a teenager, Gable was fastidious about his dress and his appearance. As a film star, his favorite recreations, duck hunting and fishing, saw Gable outfitted like an ad for Abercrombie and Fitch. Had he any detractors, not one would ever choose the word 'slob' to denigrate Clark Gable. Whether or not he really considered himself just lucky, he could not really have seen himself as a slob. His remark was an apology for not only having emerged from the State of Ohio, but from an Ohio town that could only be characterized as lower Slobovia.

American celebrities had better be born in Philadelphia, Boston, Denver, Montreal or even Toronto – best of all in New York City where the inhabitants consider that city the absolute art and cultural center of the world. Elsewhere in the State of New York is not acceptable. 'Upstate' is a curse word applied by the anointed of Manhattan to an area they feel is more remote and primitive than Dawson City.

Ohio is considered Mid-West (although geographically, it is still part of the Eastern States) and the Mid-West although acknowledged to be 'The Cradle of Presidents', is just not felt to be right as providing background and environment for the development of serious artists. Hence Gable's putting himself down as a 'slob from Ohio'.

Growing up in a ghastly place like Hopedale and somehow achieving the legendary status of Clark Gable is indeed a feat worthy of monumental recognition. And how that feat was accomplished provides even more speculative answers to the mystery of one man's having become a film star absolutely unlike any other before him – or any of his contemporaries.

Rudolph Valentino had affected thousands of women like catnip but men, for the most part, were either cool or outright hostile to his image and usually contemptuous of his uninhibited love-making techniques. John Wayne could count on legions of men who admired the rugged masculinity he projected along with the unwavering challenge he implied to the pacifist liberals of his country. But Wayne seldom became a pin-up for adoring women.

Only Clark Gable achieved the seemingly impossible in enlisting the approval of male film goers while he became the ideal man amongst men or women — women who found his sardonic good humor, often turned against himself, along with his tigerish handsomeness, a combination that brought him almost unbearingly close to fantasy fulfilling perfection.

After considering the mystery of how Hopedale could have fuelled the raw material for so exceptional a human being, one is confronted with an even greater puzzle: what motivated a youth of uninspiring Hopedale to pursue a theatrical career with Gable's obsessive determination? Surely nothing given him by his father — unless it was strong reaction against his father's constant anti-cultural stance.

William Gable was a handsome, rugged oil driller, a wandering wild-catter, hard-drinking, rough living individualist who was always determined to see that his son, 'the Kid', should not develop any 'sissified' traits whatsoever. And a life in the theatre or work in motion pictures William Gable considered no proper occupations for a he-man. William Gable had a brother who actually ran a theatre in Sharon Pennsylvania. But there is no record of young Clark's ever having met his uncle much less of having the experience of attending his uncle's establishment in Pennsylvania. In fact, Hopedale was without a theatre — not even a makeshift movie house. It was many years before one of cinema's most successful players ever saw a movie.

Were there genes from Adeline Hershelman, who tried to paint, in young Clark that militated against his father's steadfast ambition to see that his son remained a brawny hard-hat like himself? Clark's work experiences were surely leading him in that direction. With his father, he worked in oil fields. Alone, he was employed in garages, logging camps and with telephone wire crews. Reluctantly, at the age of sixteen, he had wrestled alongside his father trying to coax a living from the stubborn soil of the farm William

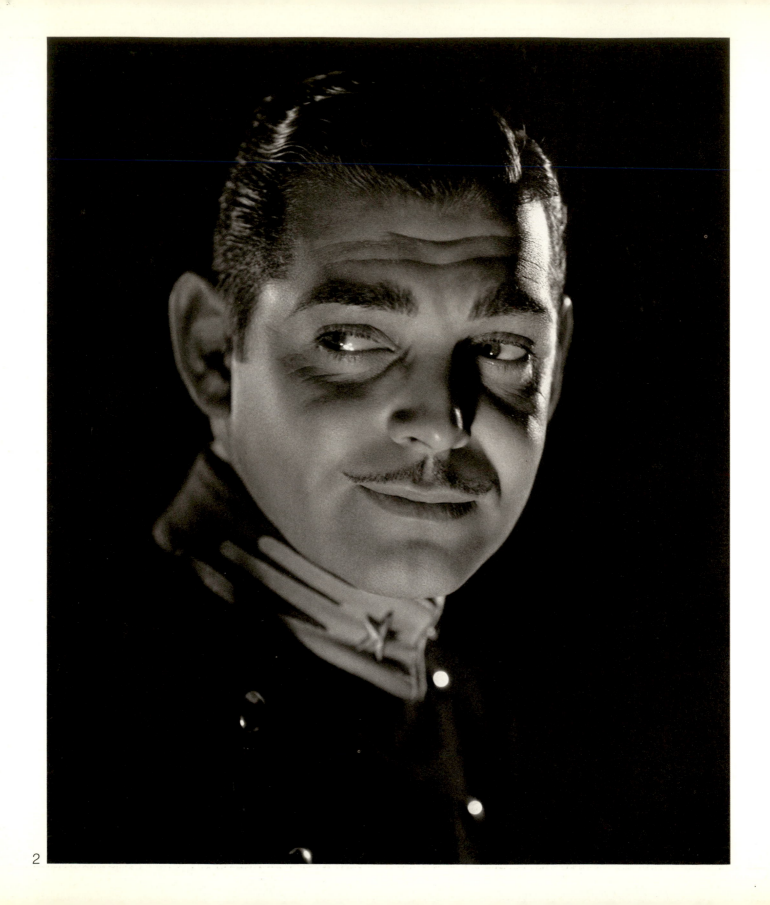

2

Gable had acquired near Ravenna Ohio after he had halted his long wandering separations from his family.

Clark Gable found loving support from his understanding stepmother who had high hopes for a stepson that to her, held much promise for exploits far beyond the depressingly limited horizons of Hopedale. She encouraged him at twelve to go to a music teacher. He learned to play the French horn and by thirteen he was playing in the town band. Growing fast, he reached six feet by the time he was fourteen. Husky and oversize, he still did not become the athlete (or the brawler) his father hoped for; running and shot-putting at the high-school track meets were casual activities that did not enlist his all-out enthusiasm.

More significantly, he did have his first taste of performance as a teenager. The high school in Hopedale could not manage such a luxury as an auditorium. School events were held in the Opera House. There Clark Gable first experienced the often addictive spell of being on stage. He sang a duet with a young lady and whatever the audience thought of his initial performance, his father's reaction was to tease him about his singing — a jokingly-serious reminder that William Gable for the rest of his life inflicted on his son, that his hopes for his offspring did not include the singing of soppy songs before an audience.

Was that 1916 flirtation with performance the planting of the seed that would later develop Clark Gable's unyielding determination to become an actor? If it was, it was never acknowledged by Gable in any of his interviews that sought the beginnings of his later formidable pursuit of a firm place in the world of theatre.

But two years later came the key event that Gable himself cited as the ignition of the constant flame of his foremost infatuation.

Attending high-school in Ravenna Ohio, Gable rebelled against any further struggle with nature in the dirt. Dropping out of school in his third year, he left home and went to nearby Akron Ohio, the rubber city where most of the tires on all the automobiles in the United States are made. The tire factories were struggling to supply the wheels of army vehicles being assembled for America's belated entry in the First World War.

Clark Gable, dining in a cheap restaurant in Akron, struck up a conversation with two actors from the Pauline MacLean Players, a stock company then presenting *The Bird*

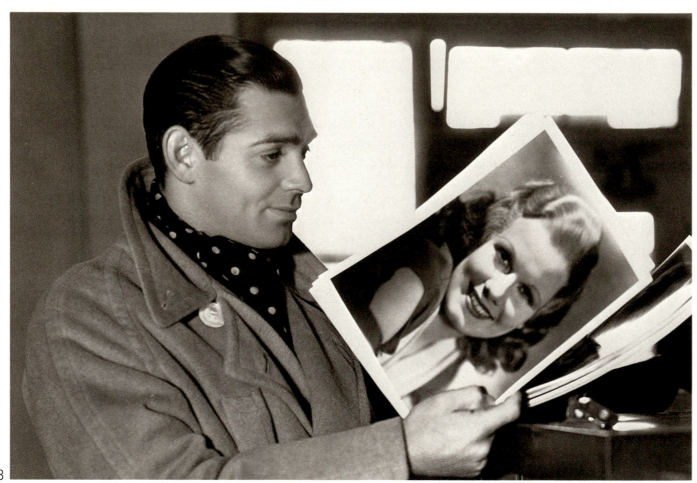

3

of Paradise. Gable was invited backstage for the performance. He described it as the most beautiful thing he had ever seen. It was that night, he later insisted that changed his life. He had to become an actor.

But haunting the stage doors of stock companies, sometimes even returning backstage as a call-boy, brought him no chance to stand before an audience again. Wandering through Oklahoma and Oregon he found a succession of rugged outdoor jobs. Until, at last, he helped his destiny to guide him closer to the theatre by taking an indoor, white collar job in Portland Oregon.

There is an early photograph of teenager Clark Gable with his friends on a return visit to Hopedale. Gable stands next to two girls and another boy; the girls and Gable's buddy are dressed just as one would expect kids in gritty Hopedale to be clad. But Clark Gable wears a snappy hat, a long overcoat and gloves. Come of age in 1922, for once the would-be Beau Brummell takes a job quite unlike anything his father had ever lured him into. He moves indoors and becomes a tie salesman in the Portland Oregon Department Store of Meir and Frank.

'A lucky slob from Ohio who happened to be in the right place at the right time' he told an interviewer. Meir and Frank's was the right place and it was a lucky time to be there for Clark Gable because at the next counter was an at-liberty actor, between shows. The actor was Earle Larimore whose aunt was Laura Hope Crews, an established actress on Broadway who would later enliven Garbo's film *Camille*. Larimore was a member of the Red Lantern Players in Portland, when he wasn't selling men's furnishings and once again Clark Gable became a stage-door johnny – not, certainly, trying to date an actress – but desperately hoping to find himself again on the boards.

When at last that hope was realized, his acting was considered abominable but his presence was ubiquitous and finally he was given a place in the Astoria Stock Company, albeit it was given most begrudgingly. With the memory of his singing role in *The Arrival of Kitty* back in Hopedale at the Opera House, he used part of the small amount he was earning selling ads and working again as a mechanic, to take singing lessons. He even dared taking a job singing in a Portland Hotel.

It was at the age of twenty-two that the stage-struck wanderer from Ohio, not considered handsome at all, appearing clumsy and inept on stage, met the woman who was to bring about the profound change in his life that would amount to a solid preparation for a successful career in the theatre. The woman was actress Josephine Dillon who had appeared in several plays in New York (without particular distinction) and was about to form a theatre group in Portland.

Dillon saw in this gawky young man with wide gaps in his teeth, out-sized hands and phenomenal ears, the magnetic promise of qualities that would later mark him apart from every other actor. Quite literally Josephine Dillon took 'The Kid' (seventeen years her junior) in hand. As a drama coach she worked with his speech and his bearing. She did what she could to improve his appearance. His tiny, spaced-out front teeth were replaced by two normal sized gold ones – to be sure a questionable improvement that required his painting them white whenever he went on stage.

The next year, 1924, Josephine Dillon went to Hollywood founding the Dillon Stock Company and an acting school. Gable followed her to California, took a part in her production of *Miss Lulu Bett* and continued his exhaustive lessons under her guidance – guidance that led him into marriage for the first time. Clark Gable and his mentor and coach were married 18 December, 1924.

As his coach, agent and wife, Josephine Dillon was tireless (according to her own accounts) in preparing her husband for the career that would separate them. Without enthusiasm – he was after a place in the theatre – Gable took a few roles in films that were still without dialogue. The first picture he appeared in, not as an extra, but as one of the credited members of the cast was Louis Gasnier's 1924 film *White Man*. Clark Gable's name was listed in the credits as the brother of the leading lady, Alice Joyce.

His appearance in *The Plastic Age* a Clara Bow vehicle brought about no gasps of excitement (as would the brief appearances of Gary Cooper in the same star's *It* and in *Wings*). Even the predatory eye of Catherine the Great as played by Pola Negri in Lubitsch's *Forbidden Paradise* did not linger with lust on the husky grenadier whose uniform Clark Gable filled out so impressively. Nor did the genius of Erich Stroheim notice in the uniformed extra Gable played in *The Merry Widow* any exceptional promise. Ironically that handsome bit player found himself ignored in the very MGM studio he would dominate for decades, lost among the extras supporting MGM's biggest superstar, John Gilbert – the star Gable would surpass and eclipse in less than ten years.

In fact, Clark Gable was not yet ready for films. He was a reluctant film actor. Whatever hopes Mrs Gable had for him crashing the studio gates were not shared by her husband. His love was directed exclusively toward the theatre and his sole ambition was Broadway. Josephine Dillon always claimed that she promised Clark Gable she would see that he achieved that goal. And to Josephine Dillon, a promise had to be kept.

In the spring of 1925 Clark Gable encountered another in the long line of perceptive women that would fuel his trip to the summit. This time the actress was a famous lady of the Theatre. None other than Jane Cowl. Gable joined her company in Los Angeles as an understudy. Miss Cowl did not have to study Mr Gable long to discover an undeniable charm and appeal that triumphed over gold teeth, outstanding ears and lessening clumsiness. Gable assumed the role of Mercutio when Jane Cowl toured a successful Juliet to Portland, Seattle and Vancouver.

At last Clark Gable was established as a professional actor – even as a Shakespearean actor! Good roles came his way. In *What Price Glory* he played Sergeant Quirt through four months. With another stock company he met another actress who responded appropriately to the Gable magnetism – Pauline Frederick played with him in her famous *Madame X*.

In 1926 he was cast in Lionel Barrymore's memorable production of *The Copperhead*. Barrymore became a firm supporter of Clark Gable. He thought that Clark had the same kind of animal aggressiveness as Jack Dempsey. There was indeed a kind of resemblance to the world-champion heavyweight fighter. Clark Gable had no lofty brow that some women like to think marks a man as being intellectual. Like Dempsey's, Gable's forehead was tigerish.

Ethnically, Clark Gable's own mother and his father were both descended from Dutch and German immigrants. When the Nazis began their depredations and some researchers claimed the Gables had formerly been Goebels, MGM panicked and had their studio publicists invent Irish ancestry for their major star. For this deception the Irish had their revenge. *Parnell* became one of Gable's few film disasters. But Clark with his jet black hair and combative profile probably inherited those features from the same Germanic group of Wendish Goths that gave the world of sport Max Schmeling.

The stage roles being played by Gable often provided him with basic characterizations

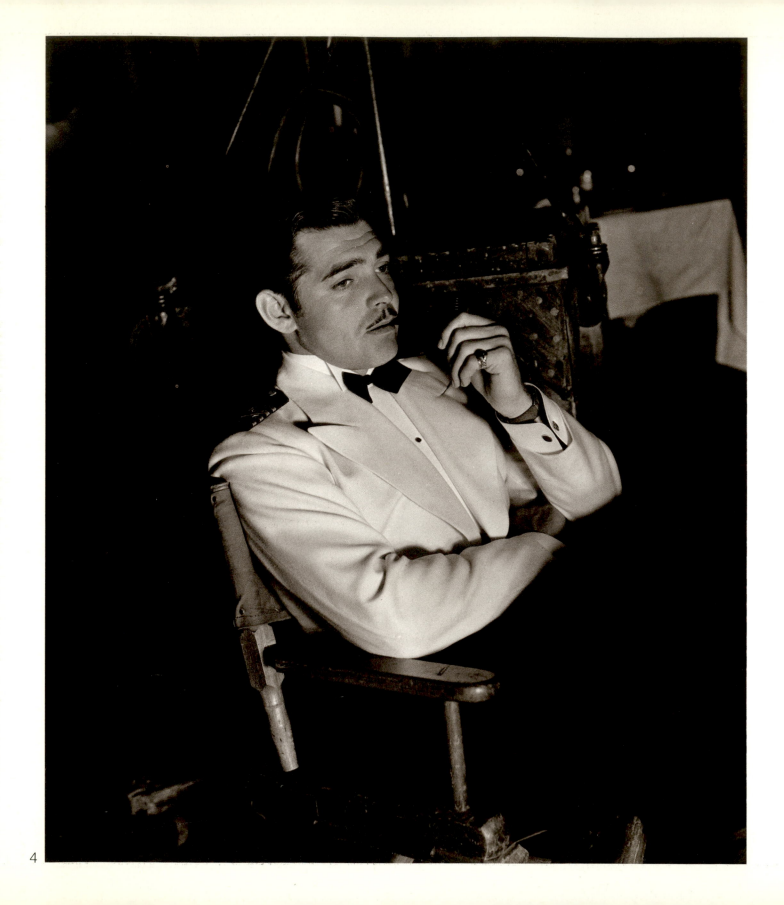

4

that he would carry successfully into film roles later on. As a reporter in *Chicago*, a play starring Nancy Carroll, he developed a character he would repeat many times in his films – notably in *It Happened One Night*. It was a portrayal eminently suited to his own personal charisma – cheeky and sardonically humorous – irreverent and with an engagingly cheerful cynicism.

1926 became a crucial year for Clark Gable in that it brought him his first unqualified success in the field of his insistent ambition and his first taste of the adoration of perhaps too many admirers along with celebrity that made him instantly lionized by the public he encountered outside the theatre. All this happened to him in Houston, Texas where he worked with the Houston Stock Company, Palace Theatre. The repertoire offered two new plays every week. When he did Matt Burke in *Anna Christie* he found a role Clark Gable was perfectly equipped to handle just as O'Neill had intended.

Among the many female worshippers Ria Langham, was the daughter of a wealthy Texas socialite. At this point all biographers of Clark Gable tell different stories. Some, ignoring the daughter's interest in Clark Gable, have her mother as one of the owners of the Houston Stock Company, boosting Gable's position. This version even claims her instrumentality in the roles he achieved in Los Angeles.

But his first wife's account is quite different. According to Josephine Dillon, while her husband basked in the warmth of his Texas fans, true to her promise to see that her progressing pupil would eventually make it on Broadway, she was in New York, doggedly selling her husband's talent where it counted most. Her steadfast efforts finally paid off. From Houston, Clark Gable went to New York where he was cast opposite Zita Johann in *Machinal*. His role was as ideal for him as Matt Burke had been. Still painting his gold teeth white, he performed on the stage with complete confidence – and success. The veteran critics of Manhattan praised him as being 'vigorous and brutally masculine'. The actor who shared his dressing room remembered him as being always 'immaculately dressed'. Gable, a slob no more, was able to impress Manhattan with the timbre of his voice and the style of his dress. Ohio was far behind. And as he had discarded his Mid-West accent and every trace of Hopedale, he decided to jettison his wife and faithful teacher. Josephine was instructed to go back West and leave the Conqueror to enjoy the spoils of his victory. The spoils turned out to be Ria Langham,

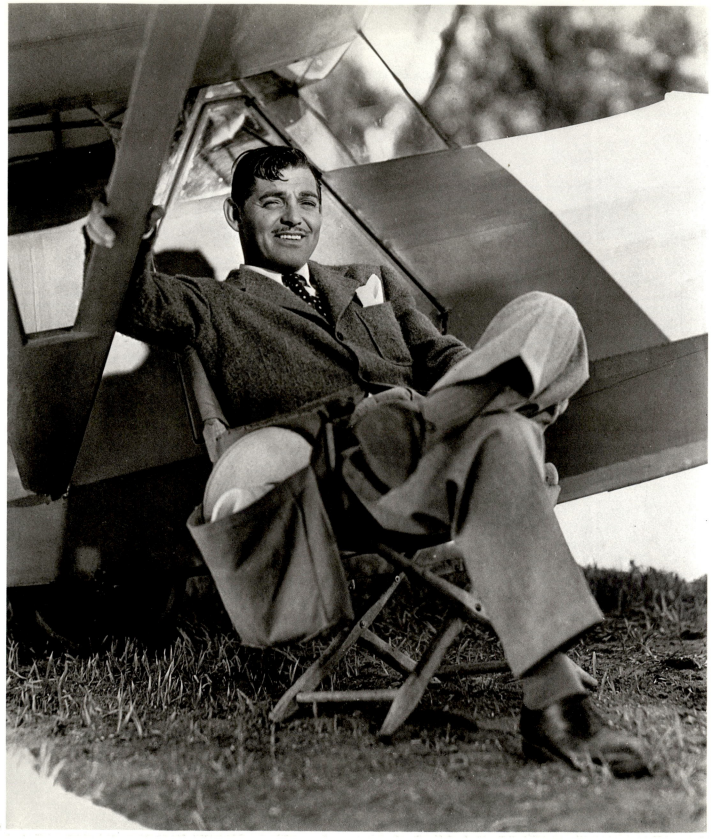

5

now a rich Texas widow with a luxurious apartment in New York, N.Y.

If there is a greater sin than ingratitude, it is surely expecting gratitude. Josephine Dillon Gable never forgave her former husband. In the coming years he would be hounded by chiding articles. MGM was blackmailed by her demands. It may be that Clark did break her heart. But she did her utmost to make him pay dearly.

Gable and the elegant, fiscally impressive Ria Langham began appearing together in Manhattan's proper places with regularity. It became obvious that his first marriage was evaporating rapidly. After *Machinal*, Gable managed to get three or four roles in lesser vehicles including one from which he had the distinction of being fired by George M. Cohen who replaced Gable with himself.

Between shows, he watched other plays along with Ria. One of them he attended moved him more than anything he'd seen since that crucial Akron production of *The Bird of Paradise*. It was *The Last Mile* in which Spencer Tracy was electrifying audiences as Killer Mears. Perhaps Gable saw that role as a supreme challenge to his ability as a dramatic actor rather than as a dramatic personality.

Meanwhile, he managed to create another biographical mystery. Sometime in 1929 or 1930 he married Ria Langham after supposedly getting a Mexican divorce. It was an alleged event that occurred before Josephine Dillon had obtained her divorce. His last Broadway role, in support of Alice Brady was, ironically enough, *Love Honor And Betray*.

When Gable was offered the role of Killer Mears in the California company of *The Last Mile*, he was at first reluctant to accept. Perhaps the later friendly but profound rivalry that developed between him and Spencer Tracy had its origin in his recognition – with some degree of envy, no doubt – of the power of Tracy's Killer Mears.

Finally he agreed to take the role but his doubts about his ability to match Tracy's performance seemed confirmed when the play opened in San Francisco and closed with no shouts of approval.

But when *The Last Mile* opened in the Belasco Theatre in Los Angeles 7 January, 1930, it was as though it were an entirely different play from the one so coolly received a short distance north. Clark Gable became an instant celebrity as Killer Mears. His triumph on the West Coast brought him the inevitable screen offers from an industry with scouts out for players who could handle the new problem that was all but over-whelming them – dialogue.

The first role he accepted in the talkies was the part of a heavy in a Western to be shot in Arizona. The film starred William Boyd who would keep his chaps and spurs on a long time in later years as Hopalong Cassidy. Before they went on location, Clark Gable took a crash course in riding from a famous wrangler, Art Wilson. Wilson was a fine instructor and Gable, a fast study. His riding in the film looks as though he'd spent years in the saddle.

The March 1931 issue of *Photoplay Magazine* on page 56 reviews MGM's *Dance Fools Dance* starring Joan Crawford. Gable was in the film, his first for MGM since *The Merry Widow*. On page 57 there is also a review of *The Painted Desert* his Western with Bill Boyd. Both reviews are highly favorable; neither one mentions Clark Gable. But Joan Crawford began giving Clark Gable the most favorable reviews. Indeed she never stopped mentioning him favorably throughout the rest of her life.

If Clark as Killer Mears had made an indelible mark with the theatre-going folk of Los Angeles, he still had to intrigue the filmgoing public. When he played the heavy in *Night Nurse*, a film for Warner Brothers, opposite Barbara Stanwyck, he still attracted no frantic following. But his work did catch the infallible eyes of Irving Thalberg at MGM. On 4 December, 1930, Thalberg signed Clark Gable to a contract that guaranteed him $33,800 a year. The theatrical career of Clark Gable was ended. His entry to the world of film had been officially declared.

Under the paternalistic worries of MGM, their new player's status as a possible bigamist had the studio more than uneasy. The moment Josephine Dillon's divorce was final, the studio had Clark Gable and Ria Langham married officially and in California.

Now Clark Gable, actor was ready for his final metamorphosis into MGM star and we arrive at the solution of the final mystery of his career – the answer to the question as to why Clark Gable should have succeeded far beyond the achievements of a Chester Morris, a John Mack Brown, a Neil Hamilton – any of the other actors who were good looking stars with a solid appearance of masculinity.

Gable brought to the studio a rugged handsomeness, and personality traits of male beastliness with a sense of humor, qualities that would define the difference between

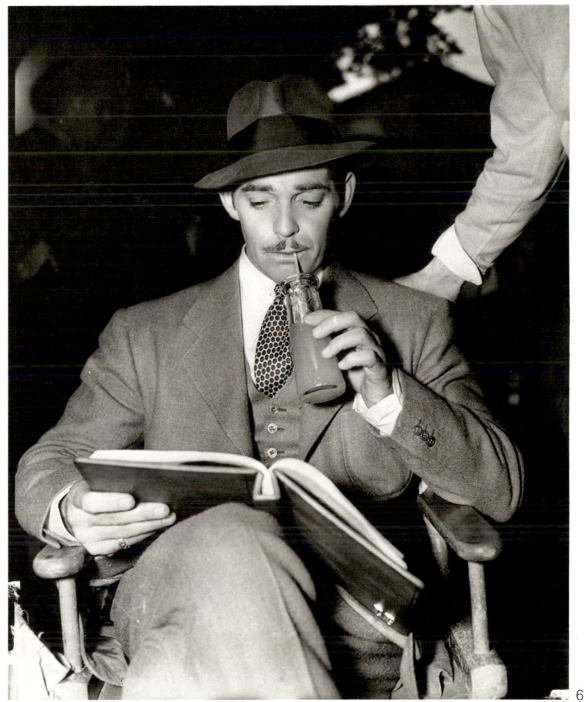

6

him and all the other film actors who possessed only some of those attributes. But for the rest, it took the careful grooming of studio experts – the make-up department, the costumers, the portrait specialists like Hurrell, C. S. Bull and above all, the magnificent cinematographers under long term contracts to MGM to turn the stage actor into an historically irresistible movie idol. It was not enough for Clark Gable to have beguiled Jane Cowl, Pauline Frederick, Josephine Dillon and Ria Langham and Adela Rogers St John (who never stopped writing his praises). Clark Gable had to be sold and shown to the film public as the man for whom every woman longs.

There could be no more painted gold teeth; his teeth were capped and ultimately replaced. There could be no more Jack Dempsey-Max Schmeling eyebrows – they had to be shaped. He had to work out constantly in the studio gym to keep his shoulders broad in relationship to a waist-line threatened by a healthy appetite for steak and booze. His reward for such annoyances: by 1931 he had top billing in *Sporting Blood* – really his own picture with no super-star to share the spotlight.

In the 30's the movies were making folk heroes of the prohibition-spawned gangsters. Every suburban American family boasted its private bootlegger to keep wine on the dinner table and gin in the family cocktail-shaker. The criminals who defied the unpopular Federal agents trying in vain to suppress a flow of alcohol were secretly cheered on by the law-unabiding citizens. Gable played more than his share of gangsters and gamblers in films like *The Secret Six, The Finger Points, Laughing Sinners*. And then came the film that brought to Clark Gable an unprecedented dimension.

A Free Soul was a major film for Norma Shearer. The wife of Irving Thalberg rated the finest supporting cast available. The cast included Lionel Barrymore – one of the earliest of the Gable admirers. But, most importantly, there was Leslie Howard.

In the 30's, Leslie Howard became just about every American's notion of what a Briton should be and sound like. Ironic certainly that Leslie Stainer was of Galician descent and his English of a quality that the Professor Higgins he later played, would have detected as scarcely Oxfordian. But even more than being the ultimate Englishman with Americans, for women who fancied they most admired men of intellectual bearing and sensitivity, with gentle, considerate love-making techniques, Leslie Howard represented close to an ideal. He was devoted beyond reason; he was poetic to the point of dying gracefully; his passion was elegantly constrained. He was, they felt, the perfect lover. Until they saw him opposite Clark Gable. They saw what the wayward, emancipated daughter played by Norma Shearer in *A Free Soul* beheld when Clark Gable as the dinner-jacketed, menacing gangster opposed the effete gentleman of Leslie Howard. Gentlemen, they decided – along with Norma Shearer – were nice but *men* like Clark Gable were what they really needed. Ironically, Leslie Howard was doomed once more to provide a target for the firepower of Clark Gable when as Ashley, he faced the machine-gun diction of Rhett Butler.

Being interviewed by David Frost, Joan Crawford once put it perhaps too bluntly. She'd been asked that of all the actors she had worked with, which one was the most exciting. Her reply was 'Clark Gable of course.' Injudiciously, Frost asked why. 'Because he had balls' she answered with candour enough to have the interchange wiped off the air. Later on, she put her opinion in writing, more discreetly. 'This magnetic man had more sheer animal magic than anyone in the world and every woman knew it.' And writing again; 'I don't believe any woman is telling the truth if she ever worked with Gable and did not feel twinges of sexual urge beyond belief, I would call her a liar.' From her first film with him, Crawford claimed she recognized his special power. 'I knew when this man walked on the set and I didn't know which door he came in, but I knew he was there. That's how great he was.'

With the release of *A Free Soul*, Gable's career rocketed. He could have gone on indefinitely playing gangsters and reporters – his career might have resembled that of arch rival and good buddy Spencer Tracy. Only one element was lacking to catapult him to the legendary status he achieved, transforming him from an enormously popular star to a national menace to the peace of mind of thousands of yearning women.

The film that supplied the missing dimension to the Gable charisma was *Men In White*. Without the dashing moustache, dressed in hospital whites and enacting a pre-Code role of surprising frankness, Gable displayed an emotion competely new to his repertoire – compassion.

Here at last was this overwhelmingly virile, handsome creature, established as being almost brutally savage in his treatment of women, behaving with a tenderness that surpassed all the gentleness of Leslie Howard or Jimmy Stewart. His sober concern for

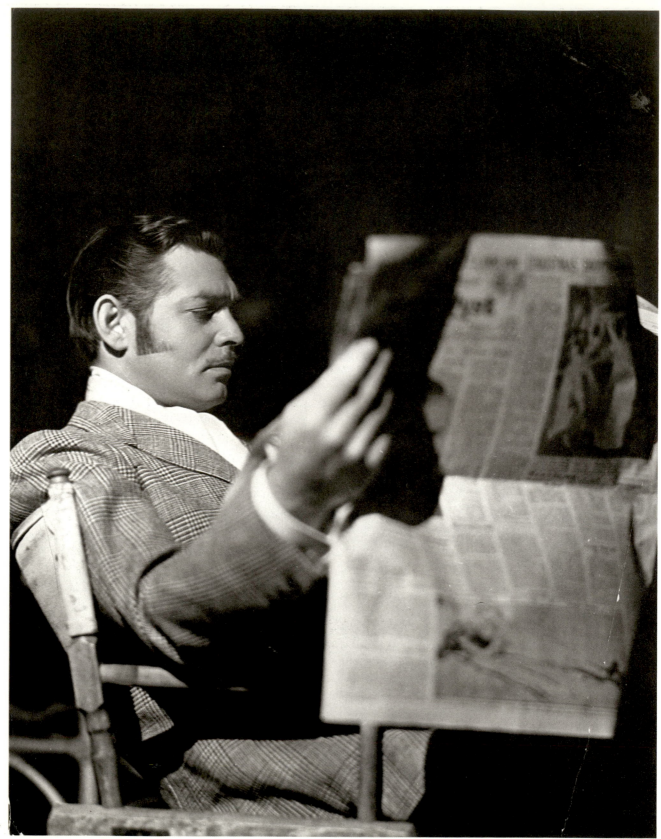

7

the nurse who finds herself pregnant by another Doctor, made Gable's charisma totally complete. Here at last in the illusory imagery of the motion picture was the ideal man – no matter what any woman's ideal of manhood might be – it had to be identical to the persona now bound up in the screen behaviour of Gable.

Many readers of *Gone With the Wind* were certain that Margaret Mitchell had created Rhett Butler deliberately in the unmistakable pattern of Clark Gable. But as Miss Mitchell pointed out herself, when she began describing Rhett Butler on paper, Clark Gable was not on view on motion picture screens though she was still writing when Gable burst forth on the screen.

What she had done in creating Rhett Butler was to construct in words the man every woman dreamed about even as they realized such a one did not exist. To everyone's amazement by the time her book was ready for publication he did exist and there was never any question but that unless Clark Gable played Rhett Butler, there could be no proper film of *Gone With the Wind*.

That *Gone With the Wind* will endure as a classic among motion pictures is uncertain. Had George Cukor remained as its director the chances of its having been a truly great film would have been mightily enhanced. Victor Fleming, good friend that he was of Clark Gable, was a competent director and an efficient one. But he lacked the ability to create the nuances of a Sternberg, or Vidor, Dreyer or Bunuel just as he lacked the epic vision of Abel Gance. Cukor did what he could in secret sessions with the ladies of the cast to evoke from them quality beyond the cardboard stereotypes that the scenario invited. There is a story one hopes is untrue, that Gable insisted on having Selznick replace George Cukor with Victor Fleming. Supposedly Gable was put off by Cukor's homosexuality. The story is not quite credible in that Cukor never exhibited overt traits of gaiety that could be calculated to upset super he-man Gable. Nor does the myth resemble any of the usual reactions of Gable who was not known for interfering with managerial authority for whatever reasons. And there is no hint of such meddling interference by Gable in Irene Mayer Selznick's account of the problems surrounding the making of *Gone With the Wind* though she does not suggest any reason for her husband's firing their good friend George Cukor in favor of Victor Fleming. The substitution remains a mystery. Two reasons might account for the shift. One was Gable's admiration of Victor Fleming who had already directed him with great success in *Red Dust*, *The White Sister*, and *Test Pilot* – roles that helped to shape and define the Gable personae, and, two, Fleming had a recognised flair for the epic without losing the human interest with films like *Treasure Island*, and *Captains Courageous* – and while Cukor was renowned as a woman's director, Selznick did not want *Gone With the Wind* to become a 'woman's' picture.

Gable took on the role of Fletcher Christian with the same reluctance that later he accepted Rhett Butler and in both cases those films along with *Red Dust* and *It Happened One Night* are likely to be the films for which Clark Gable will be best remembered.

It was in 1960 that Gable remarked to reporter Bill Davidson, 'You know this King stuff is pure bullshit.' The 'King stuff' began in 1938 – a year in which only two Gable films were released. It was the result of a newspaper poll conducted by Ed Sullivan, then a columnist on the *New York Daily News*. The contest involved having readers vote for the 'King and Queen of Hollywood'. There were twenty thousand votes that elected Clark Gable King and Myrna Loy as Queen. This was only a year after Gable's critical flop – *Parnell* – with Queen-to-Be Myrna Loy as his leading lady. And his coronation took place before *Gone With the Wind* so completely confirmed it – and re-confirmed it every time *Gone With the Wind* was revived over the years.

The Gable marriages have figured largely in the several biographies that have been attempted. Sometimes these works have been essayed by those who knew him well – his last wife, Kay Spreckels and his long-time secretary-business manager, Jean Garceau. At other times by those who never met him. These biographies never agree on rather basic points of his personal life. Did his first wife who admittedly coached and schooled him in acting technique really get him started on a Broadway theatrical career only to have him reject her completely the moment he had the lead in Arthur Hopkins' *Machinal*? She has made that claim. Or did Ria Langham arrange to have him given the role after his successful appearance in Houston as Matt in *Anna Christie*? There have been many suggestions that Gable used these two women as 'stepping stone marriages' and abandoned both the moment he achieved his goals.

A woman rejected is capable of any calumny and if the discarded ladies' accusations are true, then Clark Gable in his maturity must have done the most complete shift of character since Mr Hyde returned to being Dr Jekyll. Whatever the truth, Gable in his interviews never complained about either of his former wives, never tried to justify his leaving them, never posed for aggrieved images.

But all who knew Clark Gable and Carole Lombard agreed that with her he finally found the most completely suitable mate. With Lombard he no longer sought the mother which some psychologists claim he kept seeking in adulthood after the deprivation he suffered in the first year of his life. They point to the older women he married and the fact that he even called the younger Lombard 'Ma'.

Gable had learned stagecraft, diction and poise from wife Josephine Dillon. From Ria Langham he learned to move in wealthy social circles without clumsiness or embarrassment – for he was insecure – not only as a high school drop-out, but as an emigrant from seamy Hopedale and the son of a father who never stopped expressing his contempt for Clark's theatrical career. 'Kid, give up this silly acting and do a man's work, advised his father after Clark had bought him a comfortable home not far from Clark's own ranch – after his 'silly business' had netted him a fabulous income.

But with Carole Lombard, he found a beautiful girl – a dropout like himself – a woman who knew and spoke the language of the oil-drillers, the lumberjacks and the garage mechanics her husband had worked with. Happily at ease with Carole, the newly-anointed King chose, not his newspaper poll Queen, Myrna Loy, but rough and ready Carole Lombard to share his throne.

They were married in the spring of 1939 and it was Mrs Carole Lombard Gable who accompanied him to the resplendent premieres of *Gone With the Wind*.

His great love became a casualty of the Second World War, hurrying home to her husband on a plane she was not supposed to take, after a record-breaking bond tour.

Stunned with surely the deepest grief he had ever felt, Gable enlisted in the Air Corps. The move was widely suspected of being a publicity stunt – but only by cynical newsmen who did not know him. Gable was shaven and shorn and at the age of forty-one, as a Private, he did his basic training with inductees who were mostly eighteen, nineteen or twenty. The physical part of his officer's training course gave him no problems. But technical material to learn was tough for one unschooled beyond the tenth grade. But

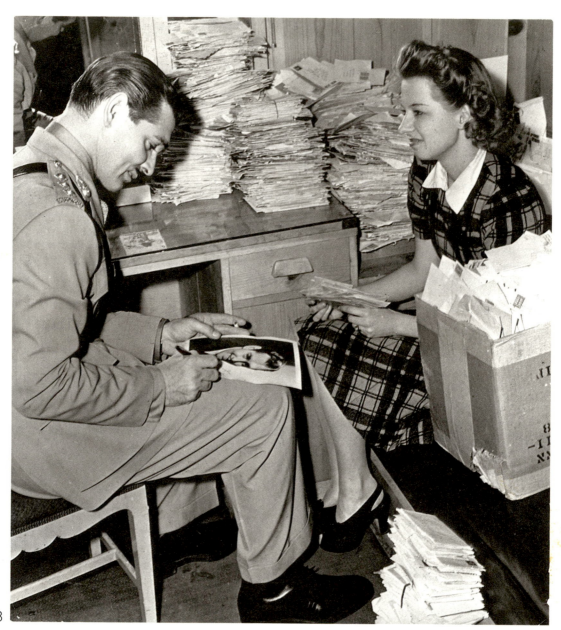

8

he made it after heroic efforts of memory cramming harking back to his Houston Texas stock company days when they were doing two plays a week.

Overseas, his fellow officers realized quite soon that Captain Gable was not participating in a studio-inspired make-believe. Armed with a 16mm Cine-Special, Captain Gable flew five missions over Germany with a price on his head offered by Goering and special instructions from Adolf Hitler who collected Gable films and longed to have the actor in person on hand – dead or alive. German gunners came close to accommodating him – they shot the heel off his boot on one of his five missions.

In 1944 Major Gable returned to Los Angeles to see to the editing of the footage he'd produced. On 12 June he was discharged with honors, by Captain Ronald Reagan.

For Clark Gable, civilian, the post-war period was bad and bleak. Although MGM was then paying him $7,500 a week, he was doing nothing to earn it. His first film after his return was released in 1945. *Adventure* with Greer Garson was his first failure since *Parnell*. He began a period of high living, hard drinking and low depressions.

For years Gable had a special entourage of extra-marital women friends – some of them appearing again and again – always available when he wanted them. Others were glamorous models and socialites. Among his regulars were Virginia Grey, Carol Gibson, Gwen Seeger. There were prominent beauties: Anita Colby and Millicent Rogers. And he was always a welcome caller at Joan Crawford's. It was a period when he became a hard-riding motorcyclist with a group of close, disaster-seeking friends.

And then he made a big mistake. There are many theories about his choice of Sylvia Ashley as his next bride. One writer supposes that he saw in her another Lombard for she was blonde, witty and effervescent and notwithstanding her marriages to no fewer than two British aristocrats, she had been a rough and tumble performer in vaudeville and night clubs, and her previous husband was Douglas Fairbanks Sr, a king in his own day.

But if her beginning had been theatrical, her life style was intended to reflect the name she bore as Lady Ashley.

There had been an earlier period in Hollywood when many members of what was considered Hollywood Royalty sought to confirm their illustrious status by marriages to genuine European titles. Gloria Swanson, Pola Negri, Constance Bennett and many others swanked about as Marquises, Countesses and Duchesses. What Anglophile Douglas Fairbanks thought he might acquire by marrying Lady Ashley thereby abandoning the established matriarch of Hollywood, Mary Pickford, is difficult to imagine. But marry her he did and revelled in a union that brought him as a frequent visitor to the estates of the likes of the Duke of Sutherland and other Lords of the Empire.

Did Gable think to class up his Hopedale beginnings by acquiring a Lady Ashley? Whatever his reasons, the marriage turned out to be a ghastly mistake. Sylvia redecorated his beloved home with taste more redolent of music halls than the estates of British nobility. Though she made a valiant attempt to follow her husband on his duck-shooting, fishing expeditions, her embarrassing imposition of flouncy decor around rugged cabins became a huge annoyance to her unhappy husband.

After a disastrous dinner party that pained Gable to the point of leaving his guests and hiding in his room, he had enough. Once again, the charge of heartlessness could be laid at his door as he ended his marriage with little ceremony but impressive settlement.

Threading through the multitudinous affairs and impermanent attachments of Clark Gable, one begins to wonder. Here was a man pursued to the point of harassment by literally thousands of adoring women. Without glancing back at them, he engaged in his own pursuit of seemingly countless females, many of them so much older than himself many so moderately attractive that his closest friends began to wonder what it was with him.

Could he have been actually a victim of Don Juanism, beset by insecurities that drove him to seek out women who would expect nothing from him but be profoundly grateful for whatever he was willing or able to give them?

In spite of the constant and glowing testimonials of Miss Crawford, there were cited some episodes of sexual embarrassment that may or may not have had foundation in fact. But the idea is ironic: Clark Gable, the absolute embodiment of sensual virility, longed for and physically hunted by hundreds of hungry women while he himself rushed about in a search for undemanding, impermanent attachments.

In his last marriage, he found a lovely woman who did not shrink from becoming to him, as much as one possibly could, a substitute Carole Lombard. Everything she did,

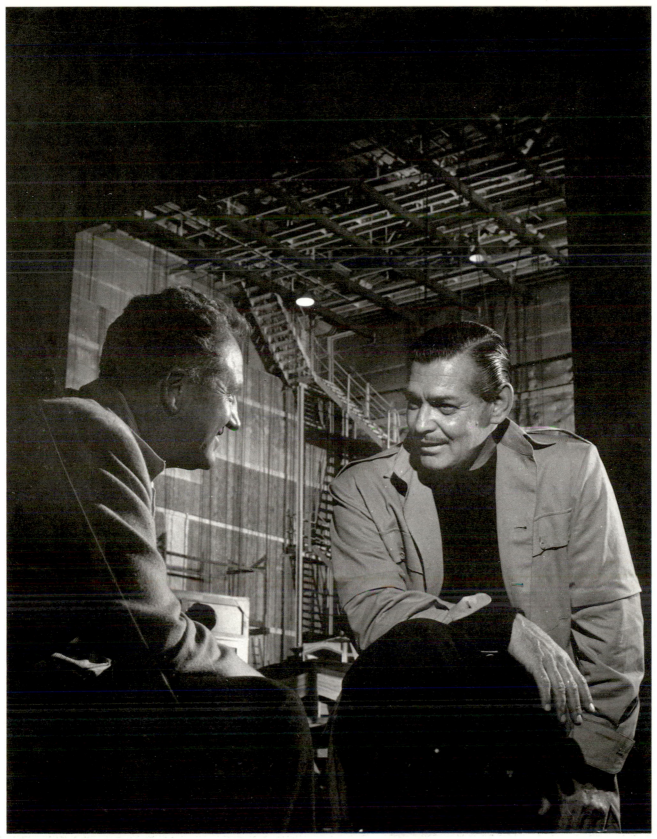

9

she did for Clark. She shot ducks and caught fish. She roughed it in his favorite places and did not paint the rooms of his home in shocking pink. She came to him with a ready-made family – two children he enjoyed – and best of all – she bore him a son – albeit too late. He died before his son was born.

But to delve about in the insoluble mysteries of Clark Gable's private life is wholly irrelevant. For the medium of motion pictures is one of illusion. It consists of shadows of images that don't even really move – we only imagine them moving. It is all fantasy and magic – trickery of the optic nerve and emotion that lingers in the central nervous system. Our response to film is akin to our emotional enjoyment of music. And the echoing and re-echoing contribution of Clark Gable is that his shadow on the screen is able to evoke the most overpowering – the most vibrant and sensual of all our dreams of splendid manhood.

In this day of the microchip and computer, there are those who have written confidently that given the right programming, a computer will be able to construct a sure-fire block-buster, a multi-million dollar grossing film script. Maybe so. But that computerized Academy Award winning script may yet appear. What we can be sure will not appear in human form or in any robotized replicant, is Clark Gable – he was unique to our own time.

JAMES CARD

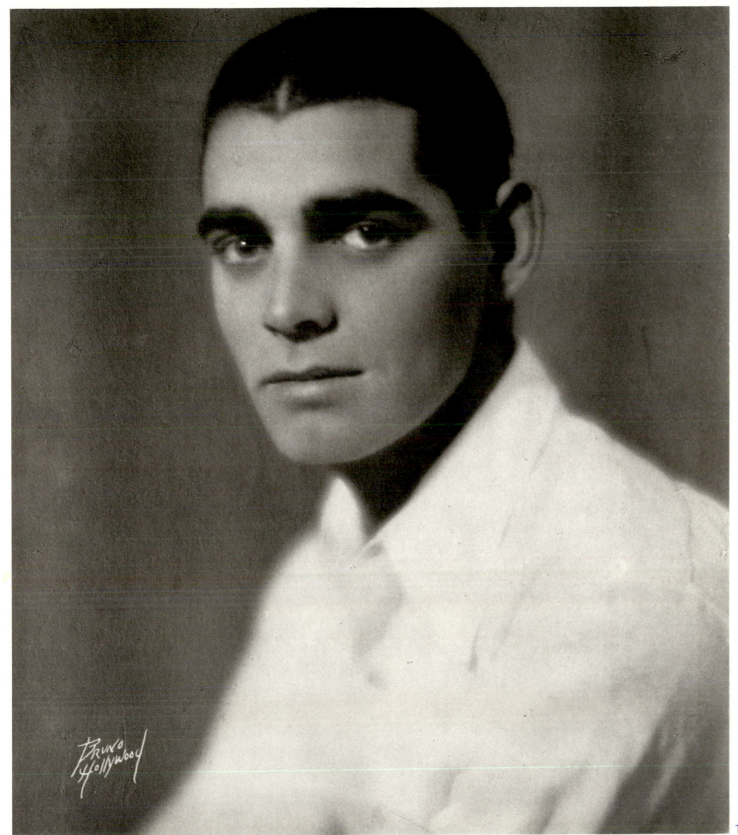

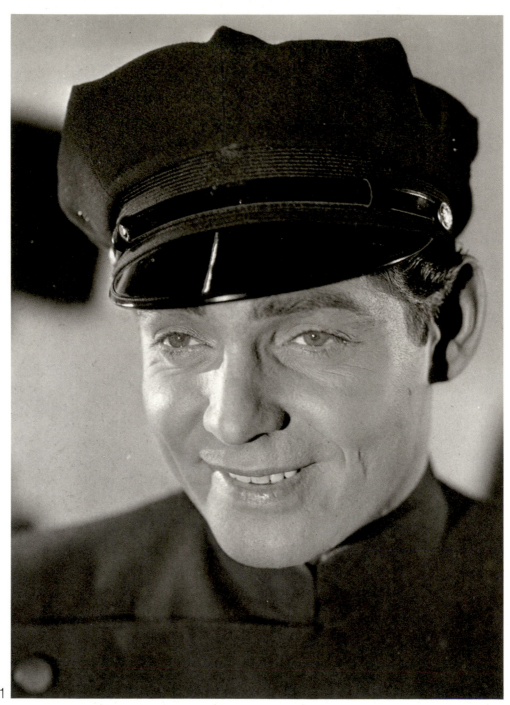

11

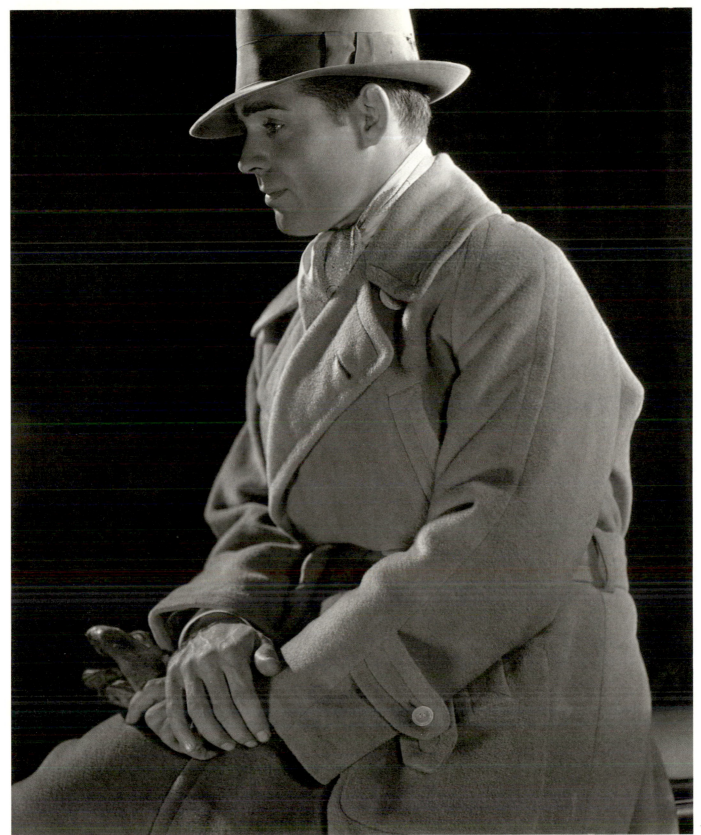

12

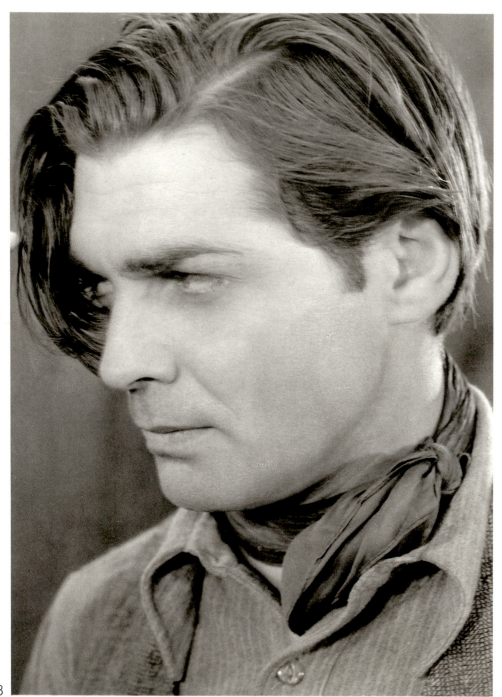

13

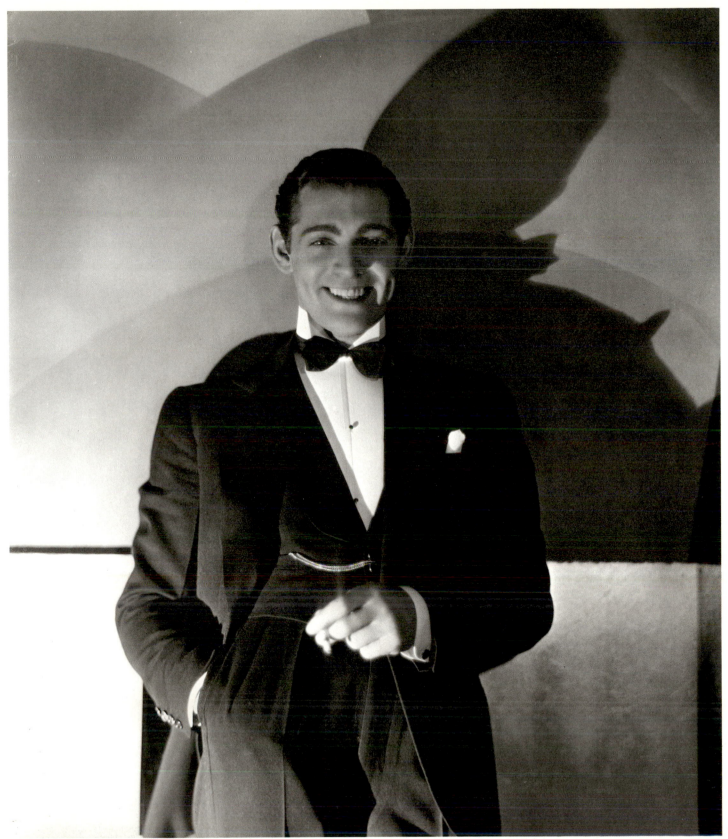

16

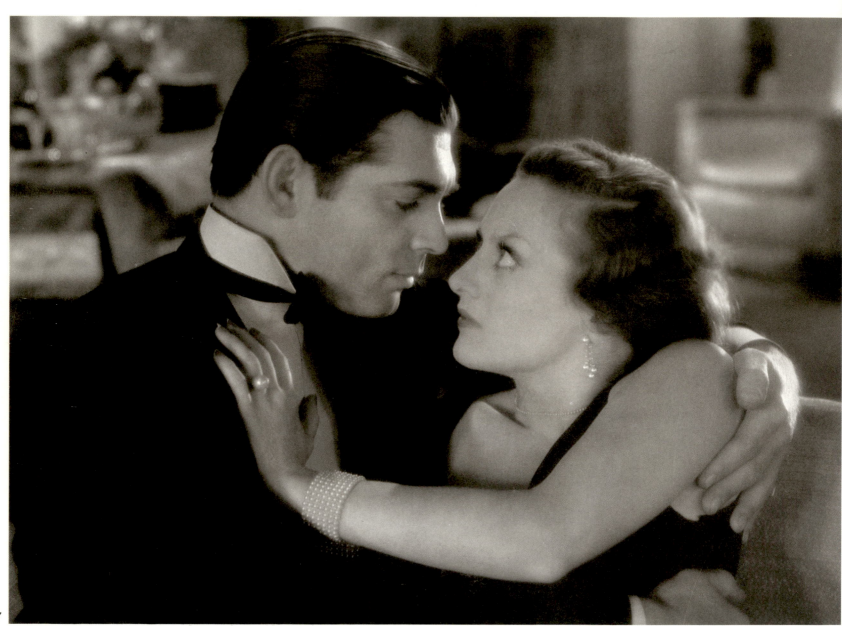

17

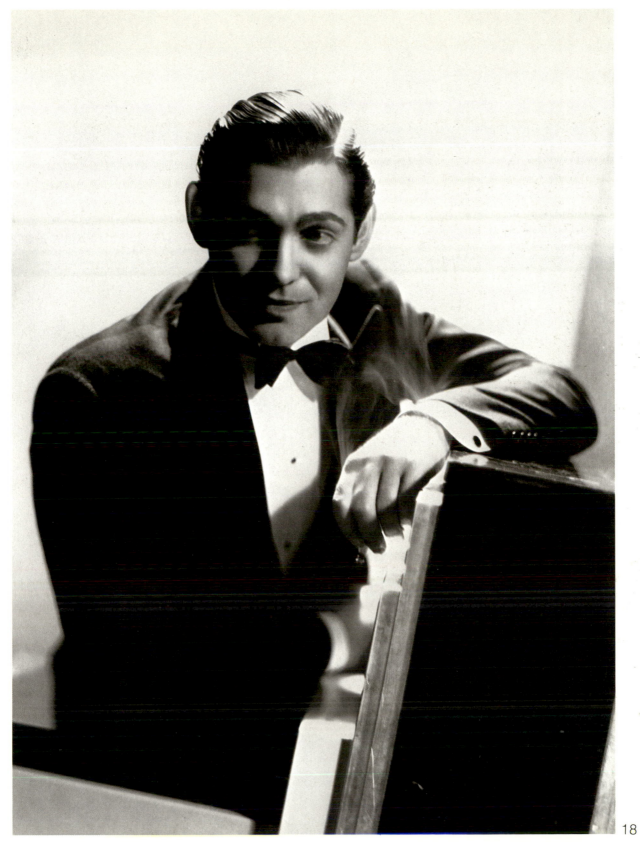

18

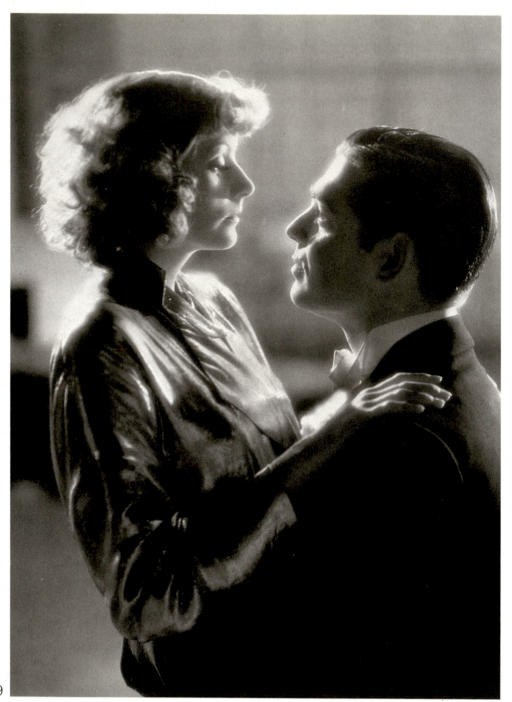

19

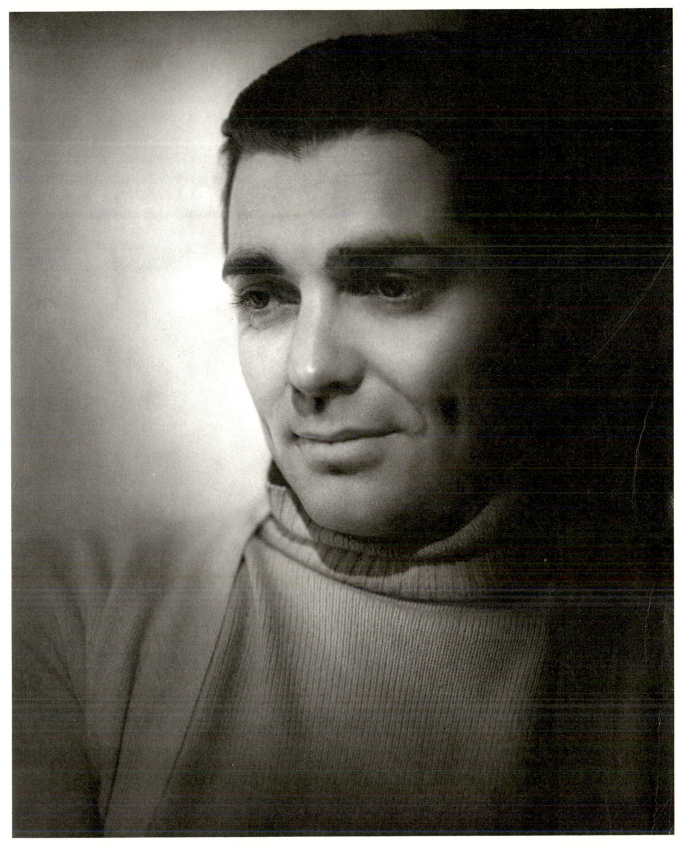

20

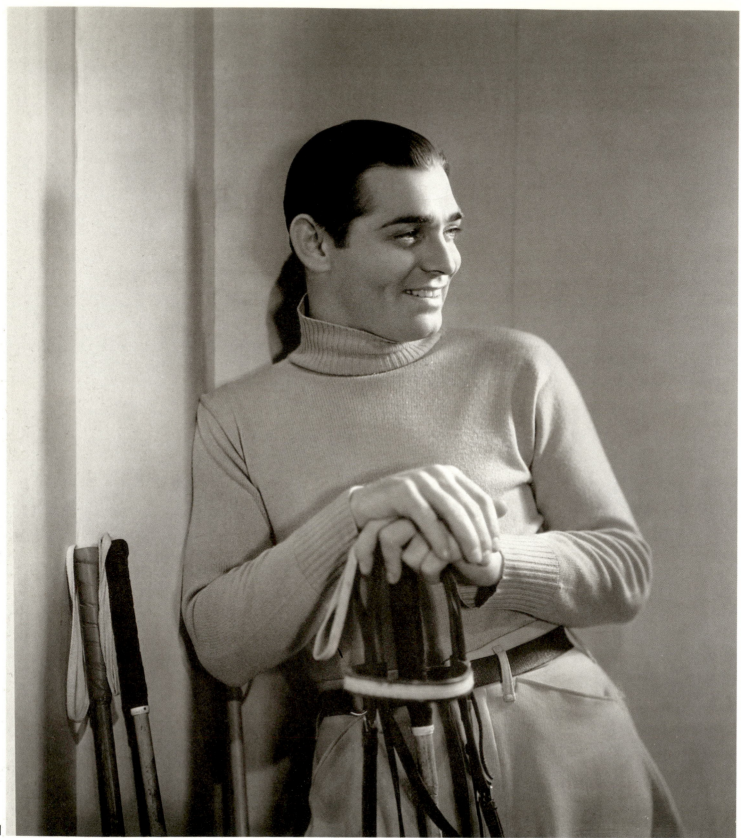

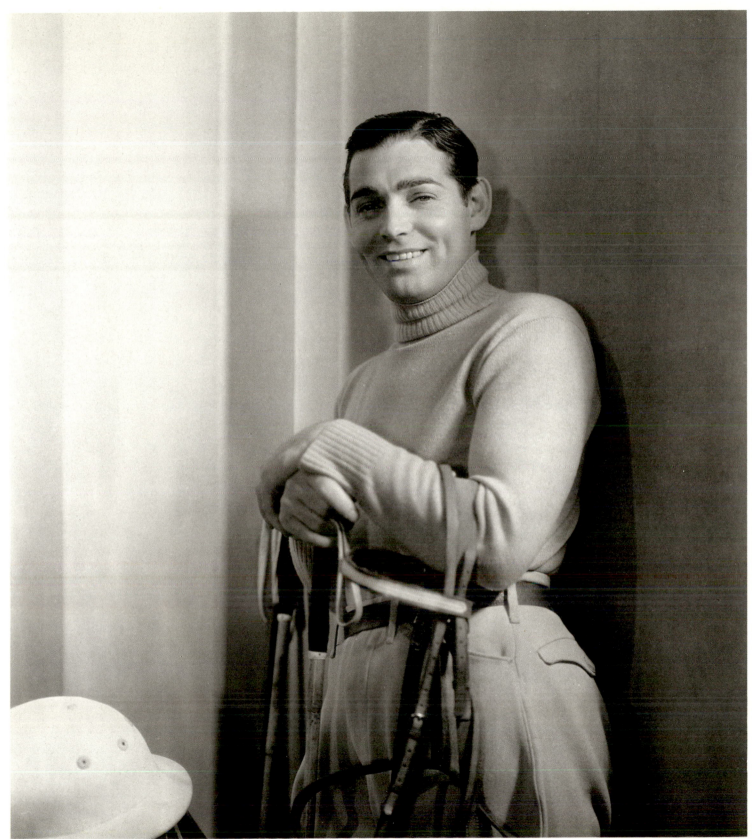

22

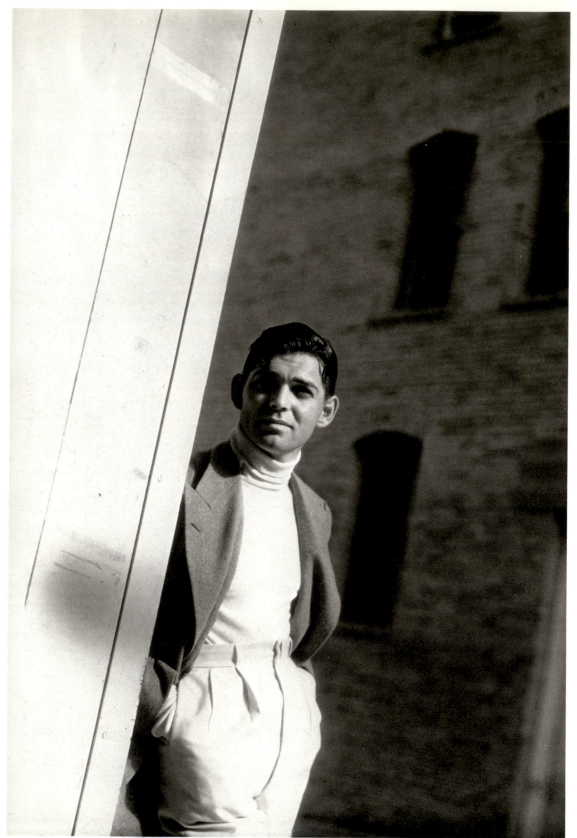

23

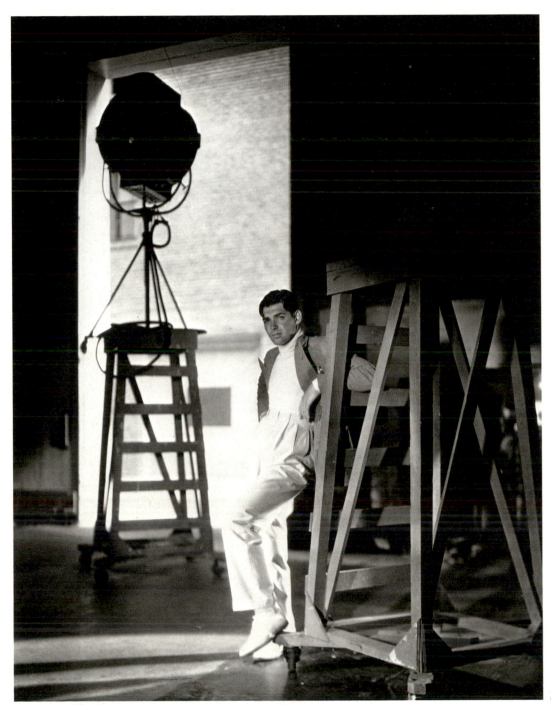

24

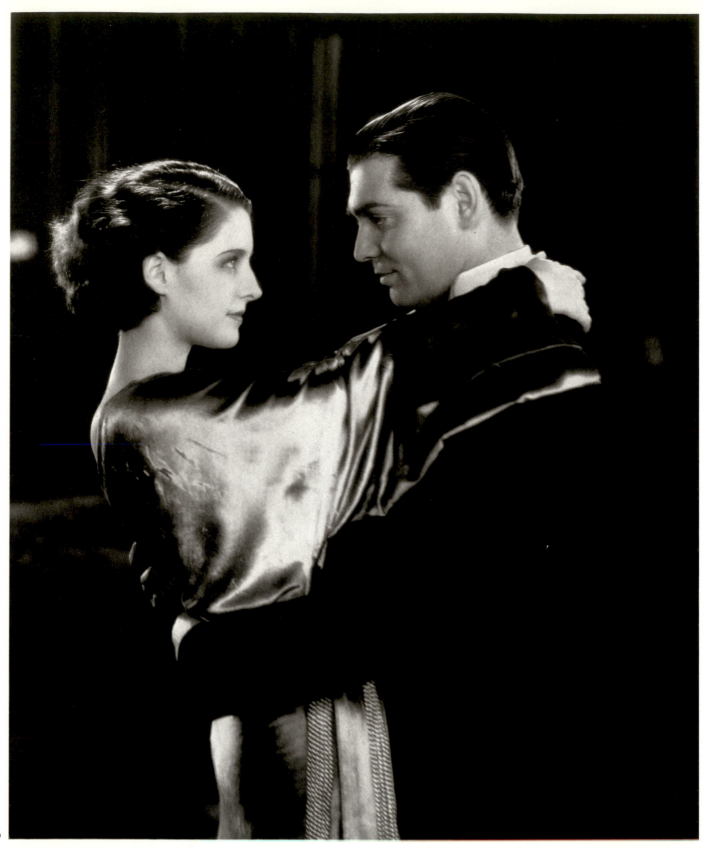

25

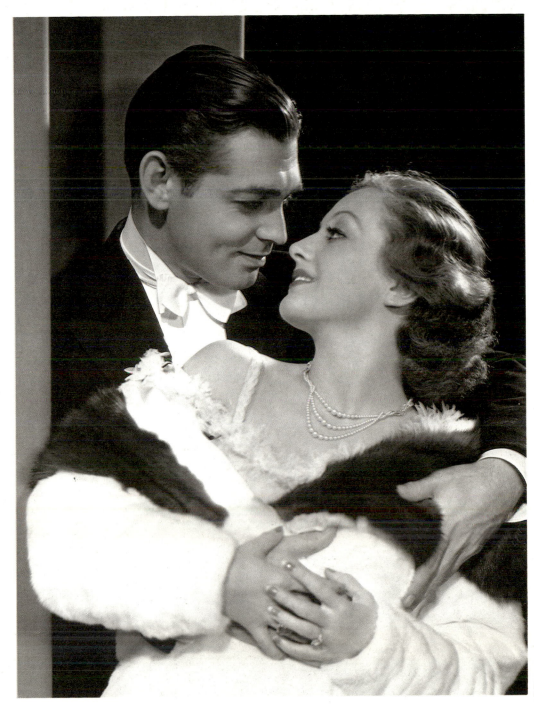

26

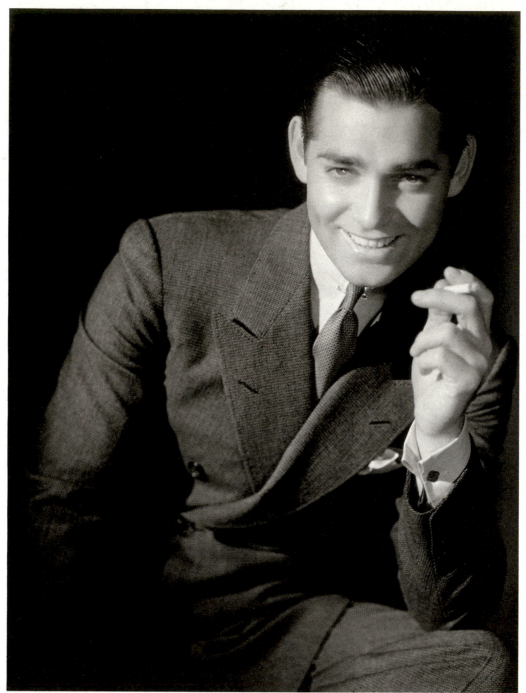

27

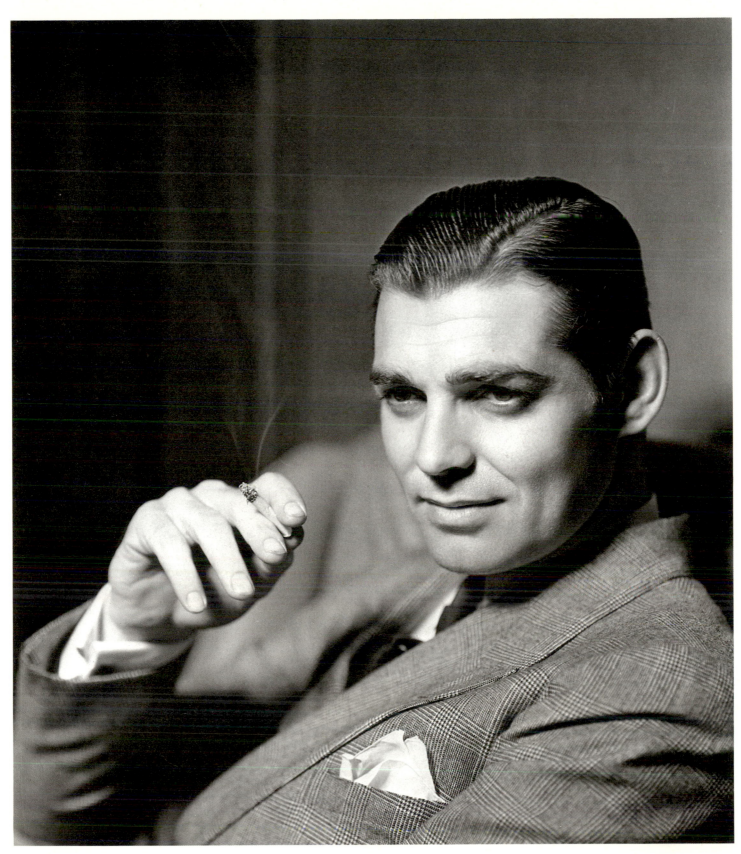

28

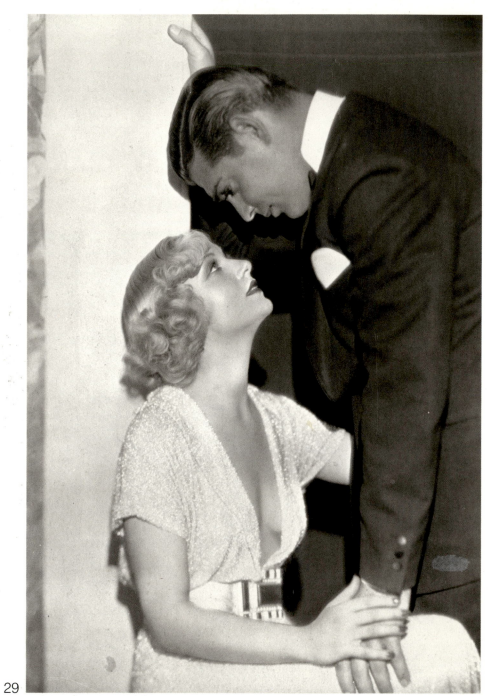

29

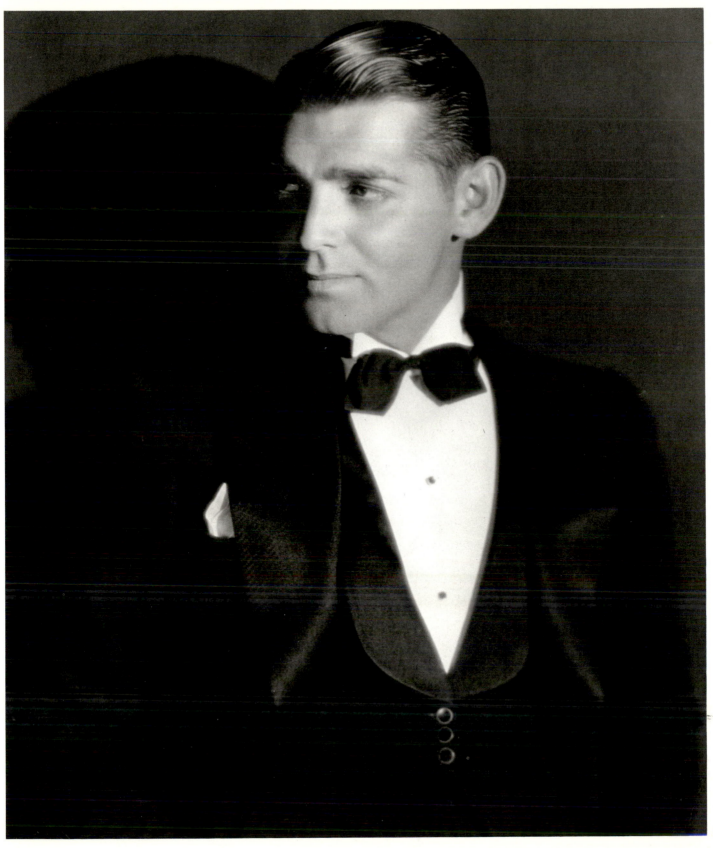

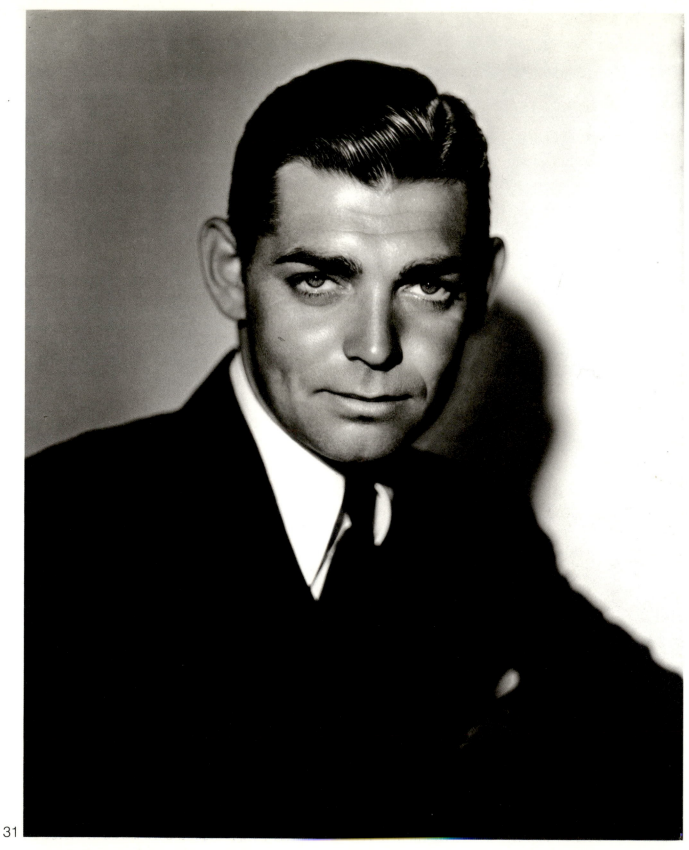

31

'Why do you throw $500 of our money on a test for that big ape? Didn't you see those big ears when you talked to him? And those big feet and hands, not to mention that ugly face of his?'

Jack Warner
reacting to Clark Gable's screen test, 1930

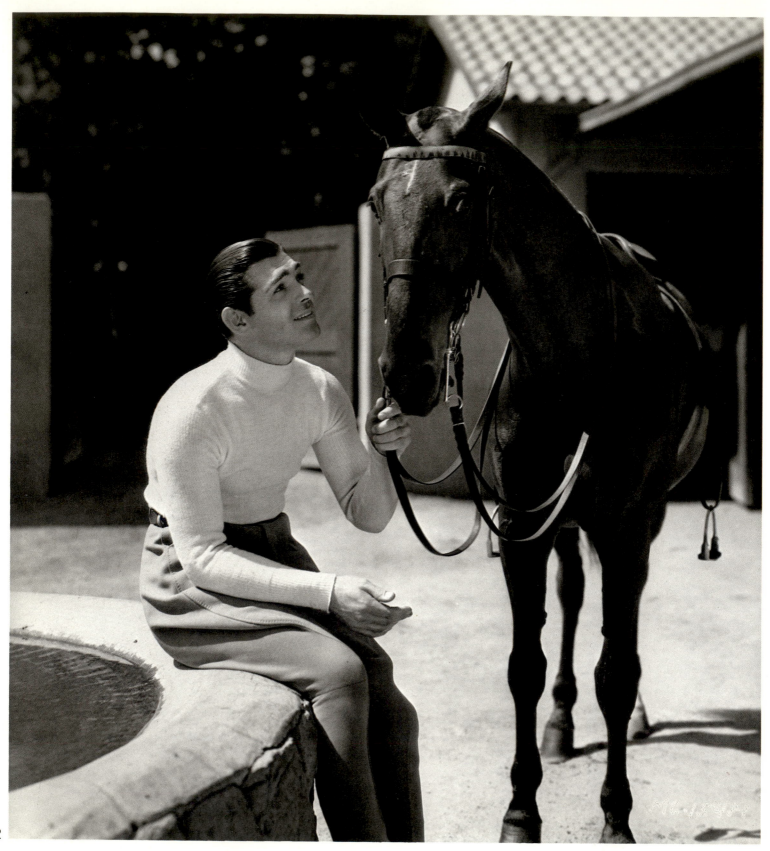

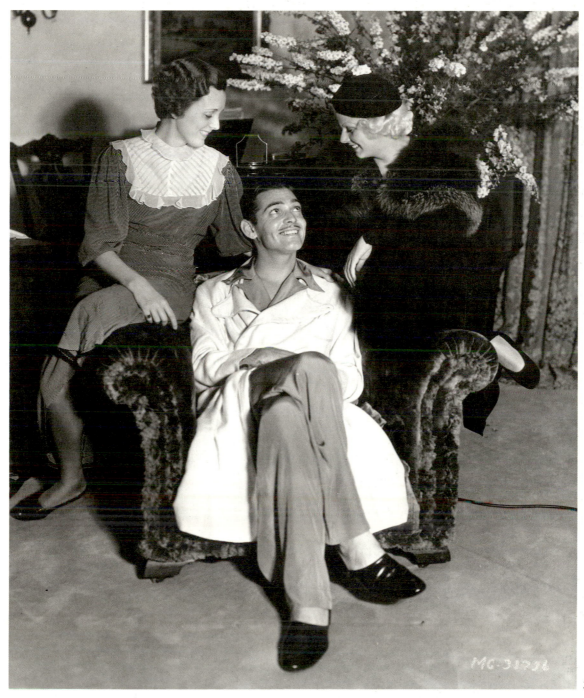

MG-31736

33

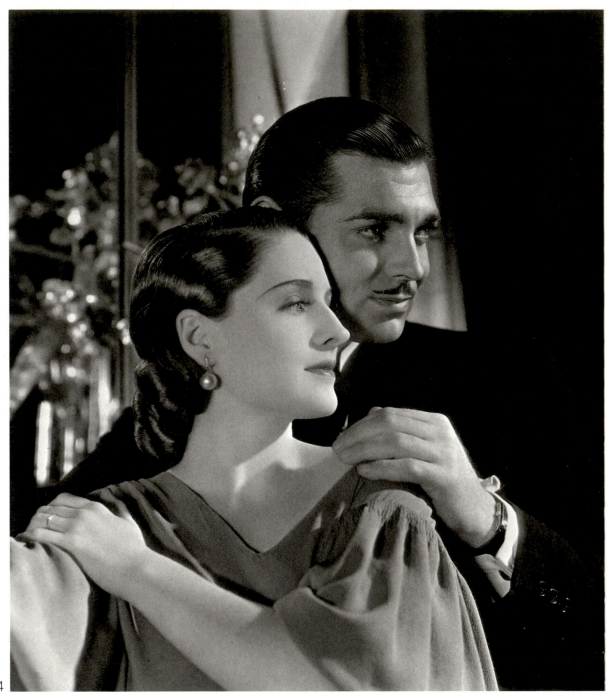

34

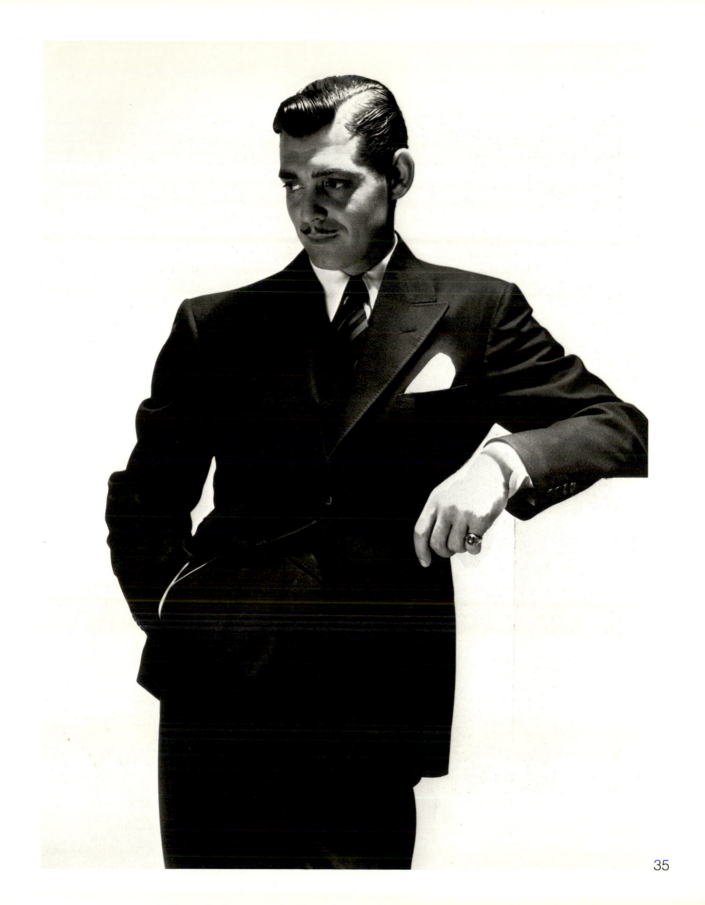

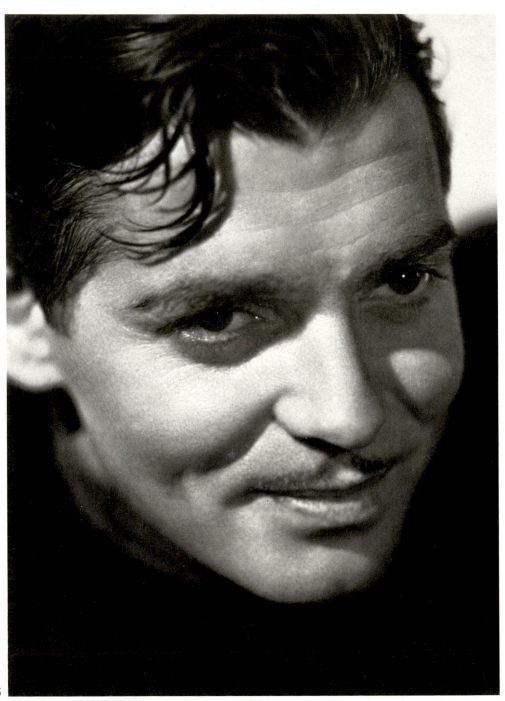

36

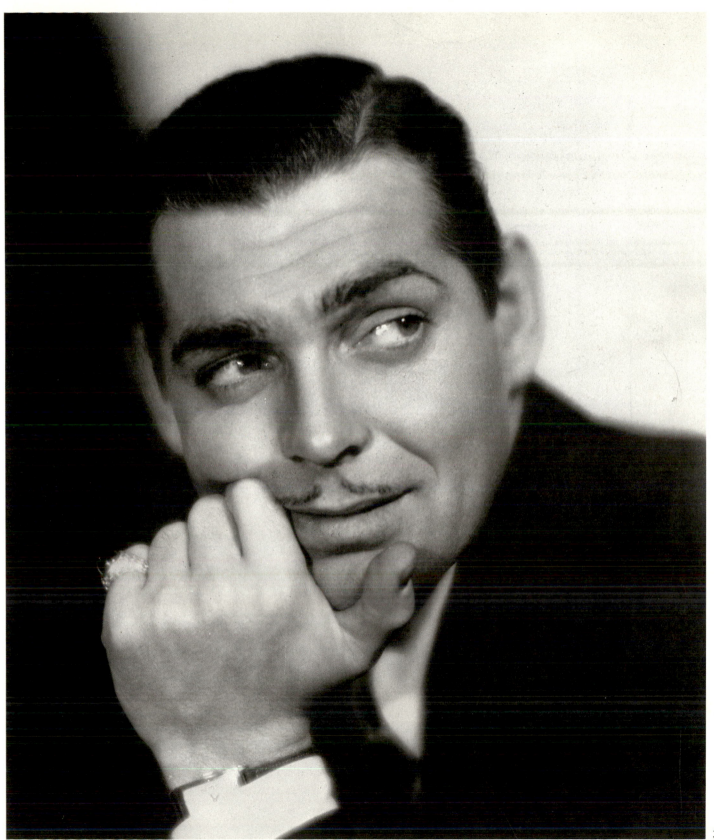

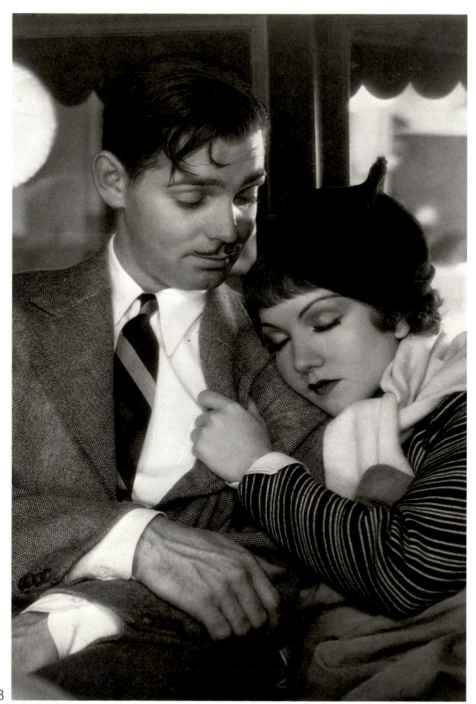

38

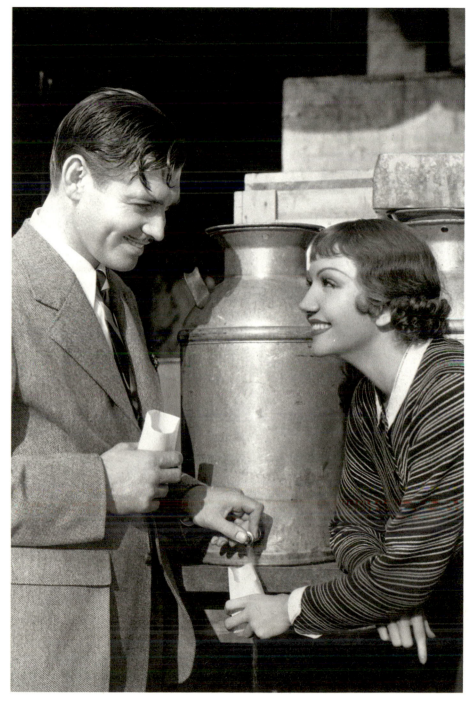

39

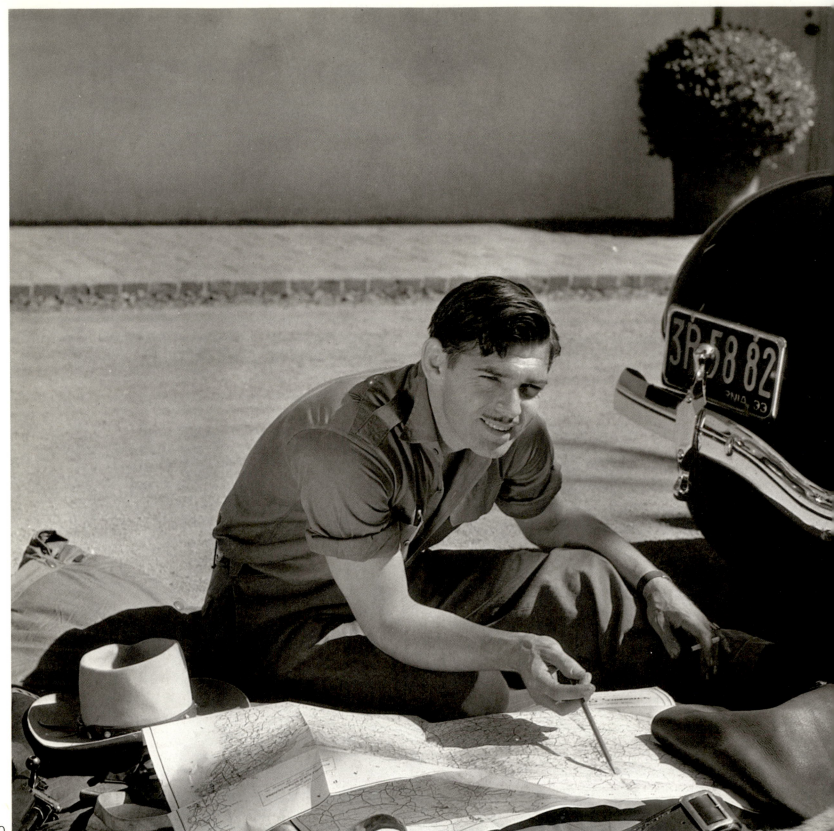

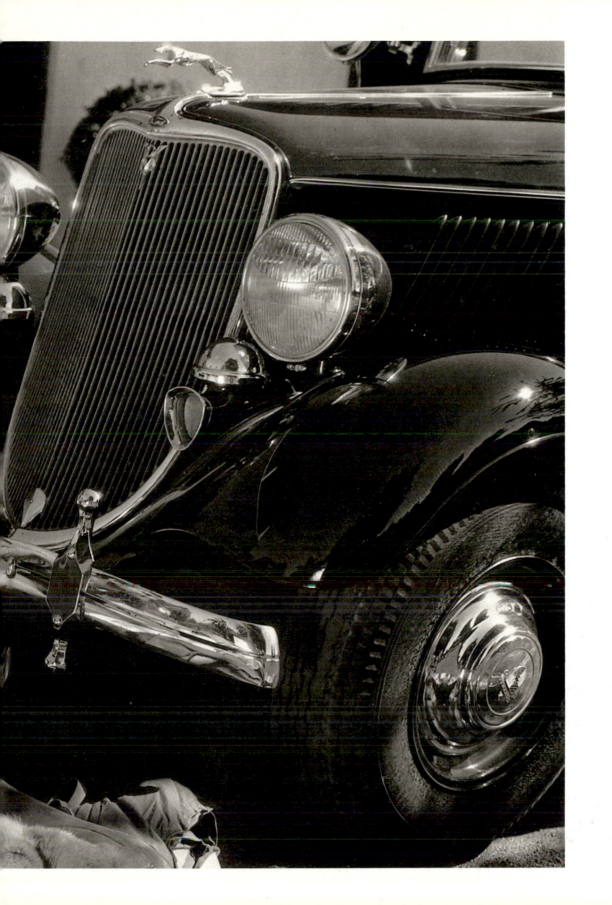

'A lumberjack in evening clothes, the answer to 10 million maidens' prayers, a big kid playing with fireworks, wants to quit work while young and travel, hates wing collars and patent leather shoes, never wears buttonaires, golfs and swims, wears old sweaters and flannel trousers, smokes a pipe and needs a new one, born lazy and admits it, six-foot-one and all muscle, weighs almost 200 pounds in the bathtub, thinks he ought to duck stardom, likes his steaks rare. (He would!) Likes to write left-handed but isn't. 'How'm I doing?' his favourite greeting. Hides behind the set when powdering his make-up, shaves himself with a straight razor and always nicks his chin, hasn't gotten over blushing, especially enjoyed working with Garbo, would like a million dollars.'

Screenland, January 1932

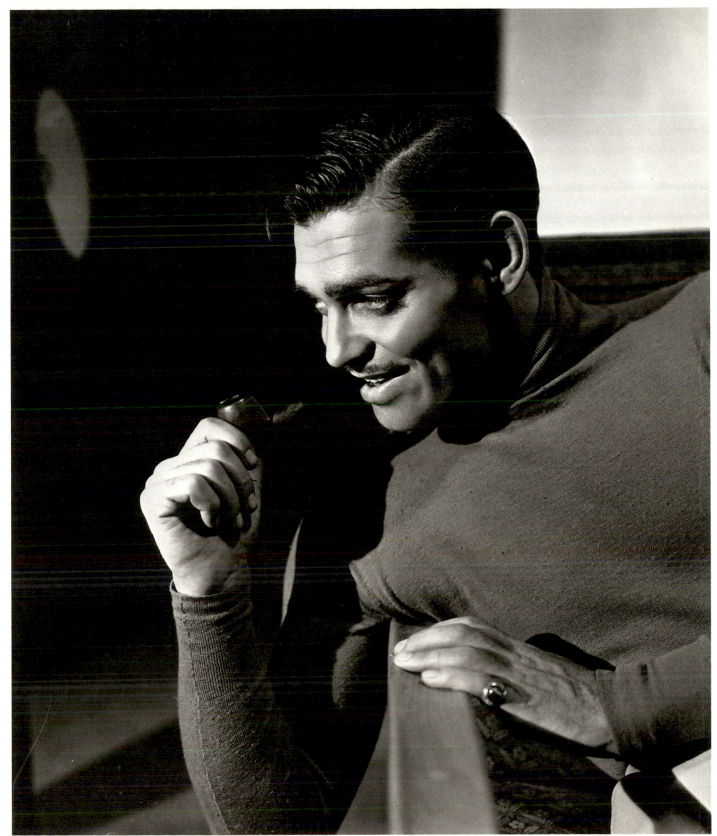

41

'A star in the making has been made. A star that, to our reckoning, will outdraw every other star pictures has developed. Never have we seen audiences work themselves into such enthusiasm as when Gable walks on the screen.'

The Hollywood Reporter, 1931

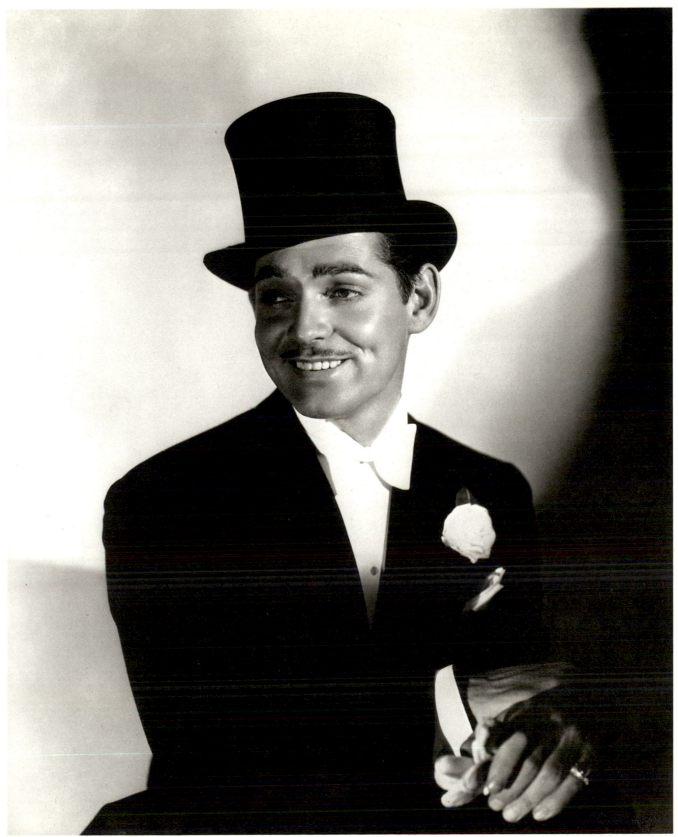

44

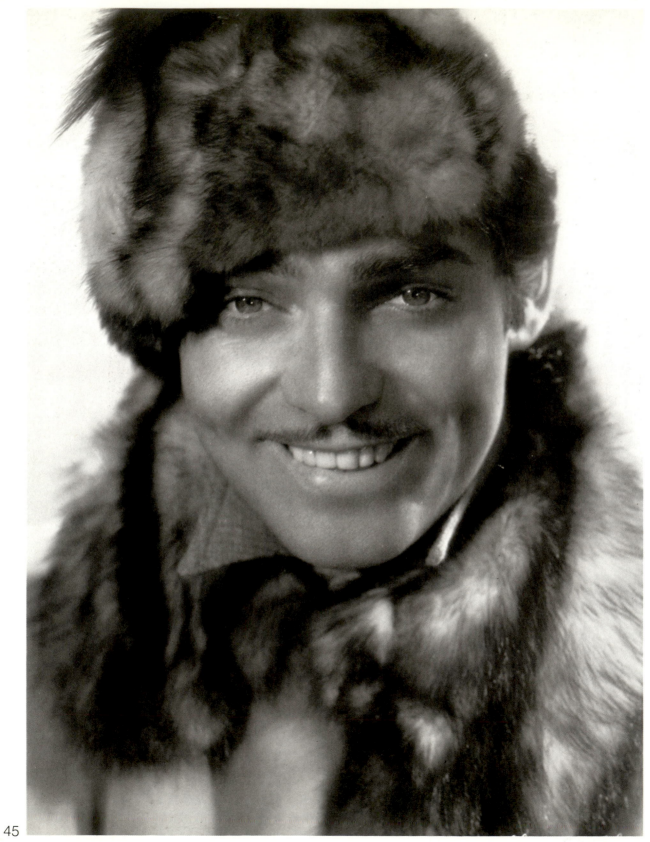

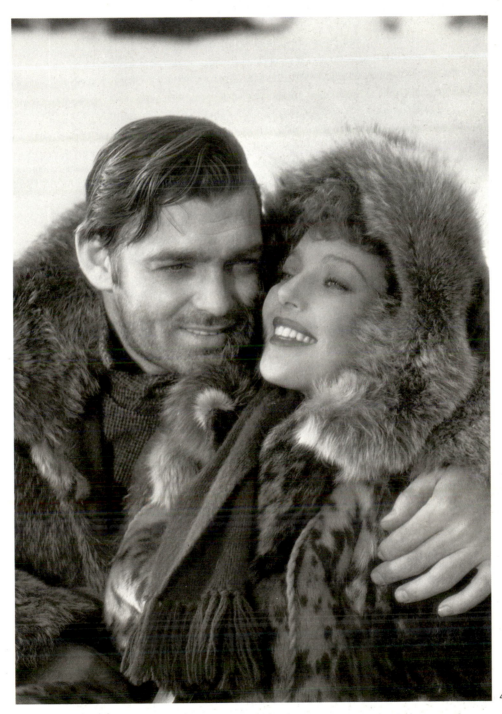

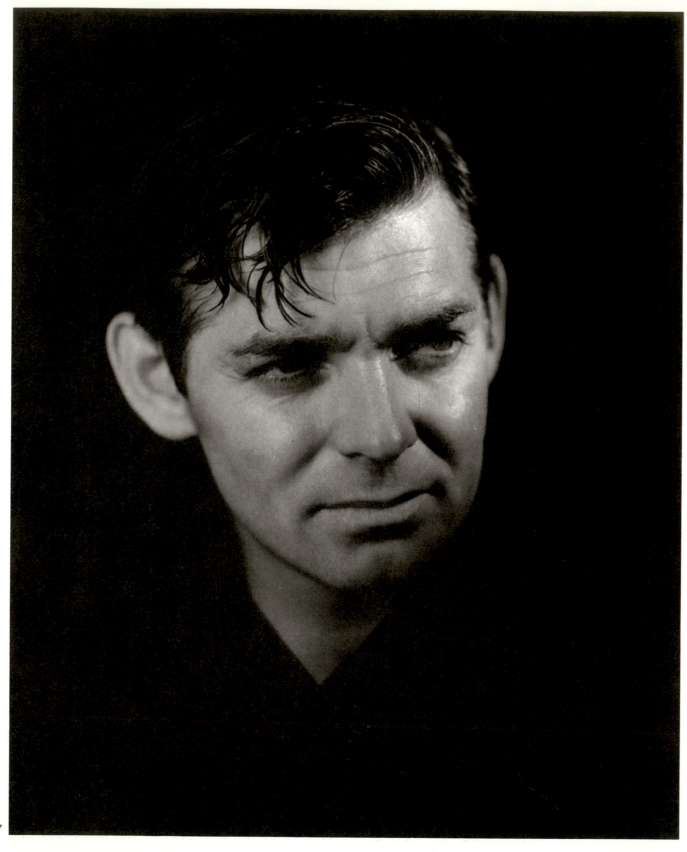

47

'Up on the screen, he was a buffalo type who would bust through doors, but innately he was a gentleman – kind, thoughtful and tender . . . Inside he was a gentle man in every sense of the word.'

Delmer Daves,
director of *Never Let Me Go,* 1953

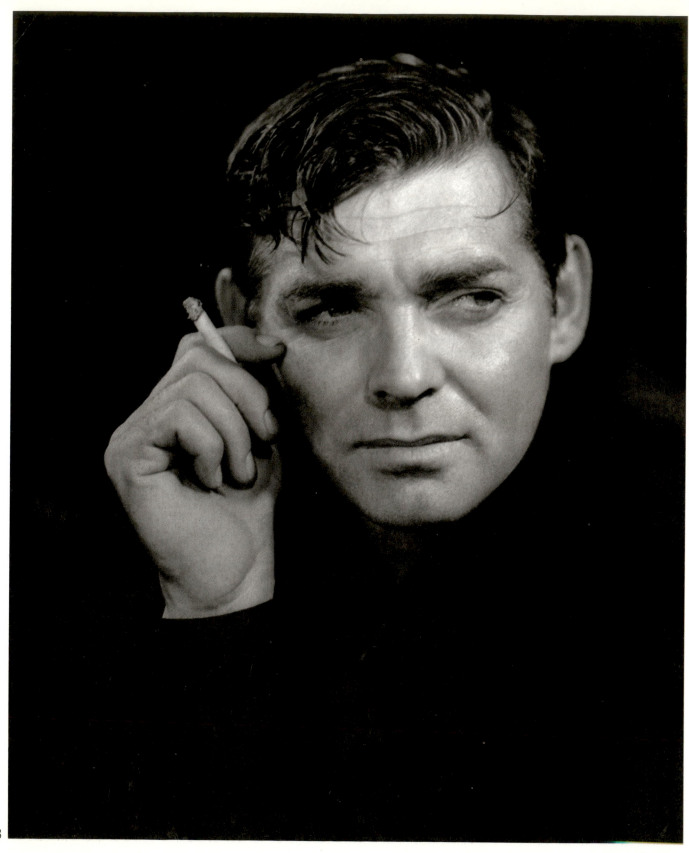

48

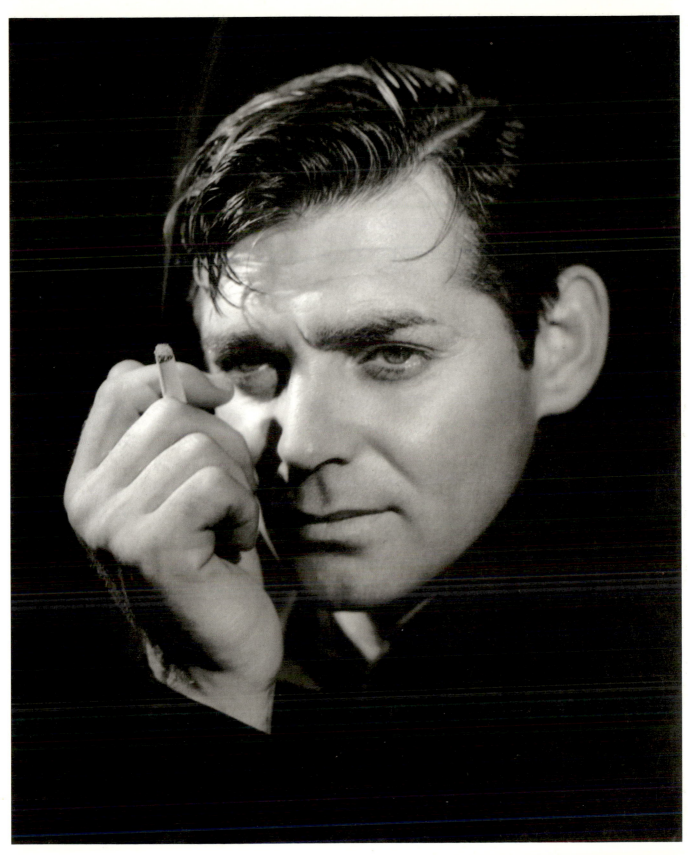

49

'During the year I've been in films I have been in twelve pictures. I have played a cowboy, a milkman, a chauffeur, several gangsters, a newspaper reporter, a marine aviator, a plain bum, practically everything.

And during these months I have grown to like pictures. Today I think of nothing else. I am afraid of rapid success. It is so easy to stick a pin in a balloon. It worries me. I have been broke too often, broke and stranded, I have seen my hopes built up and dashed down too often, to have any illusions of quick success.'

Clark Gable, 1931

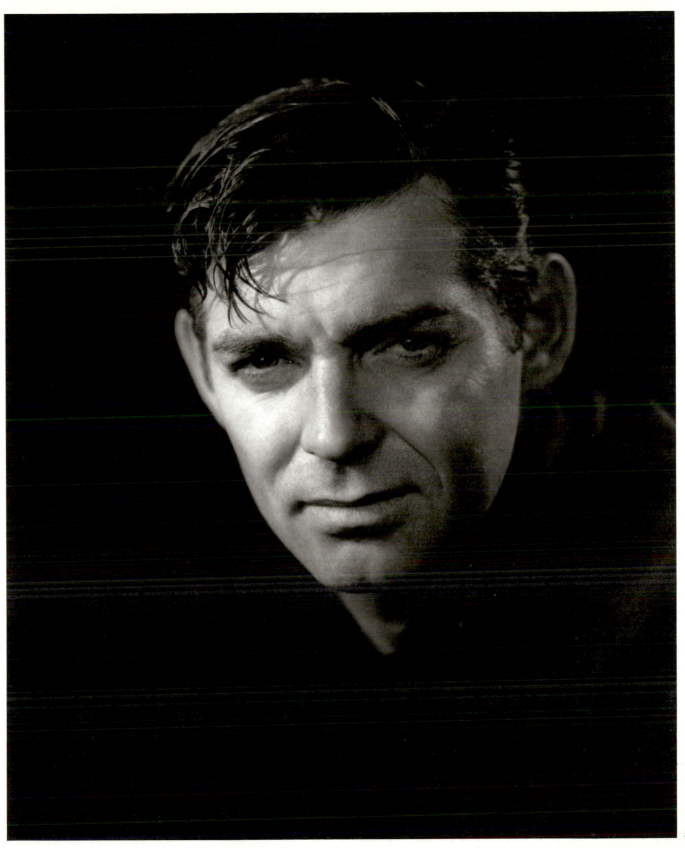

50

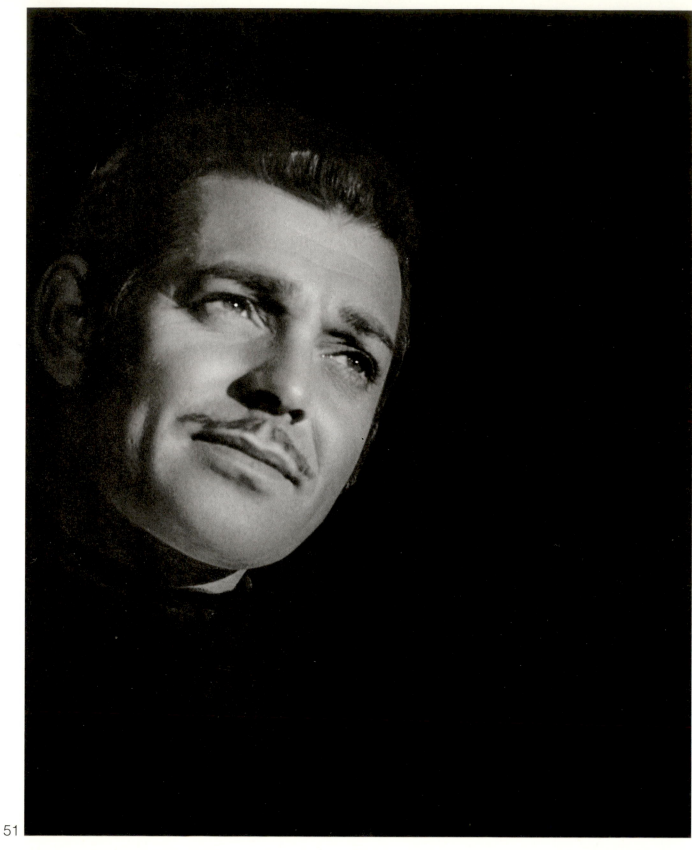

51

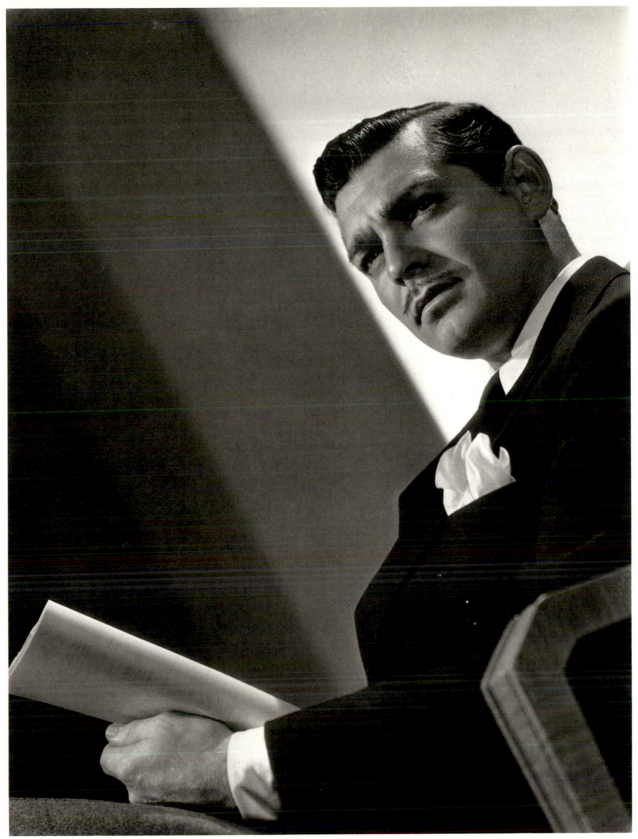

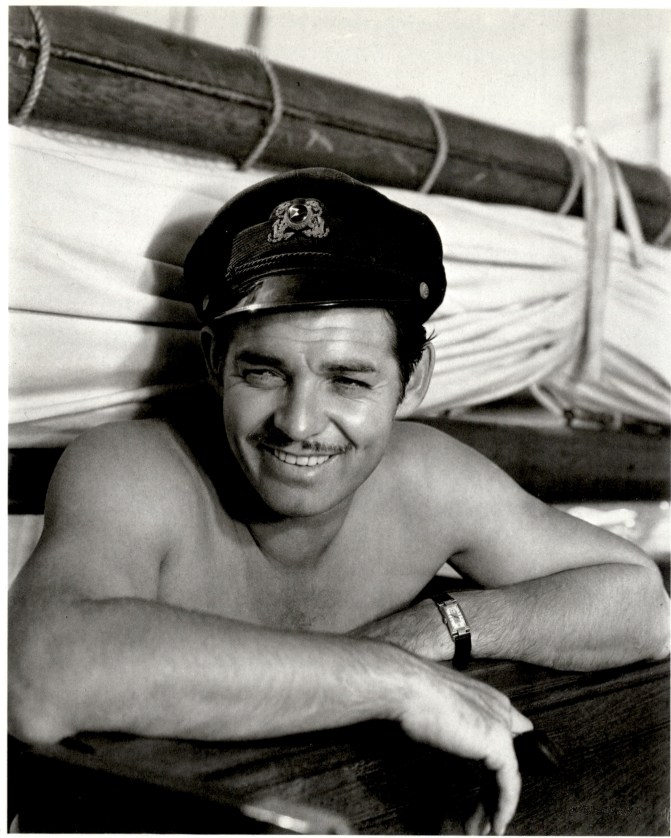

53

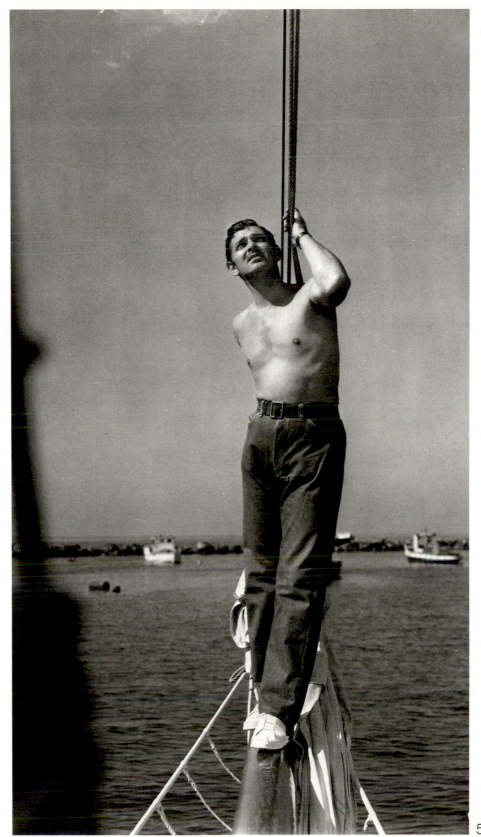

54

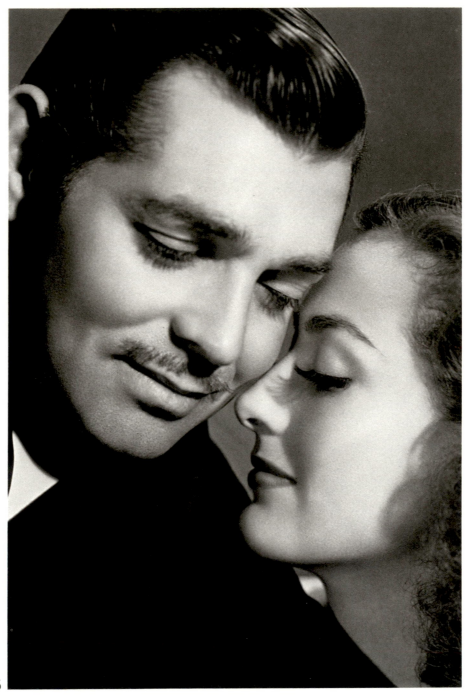

55

'My God you're big!'

Joan Crawford

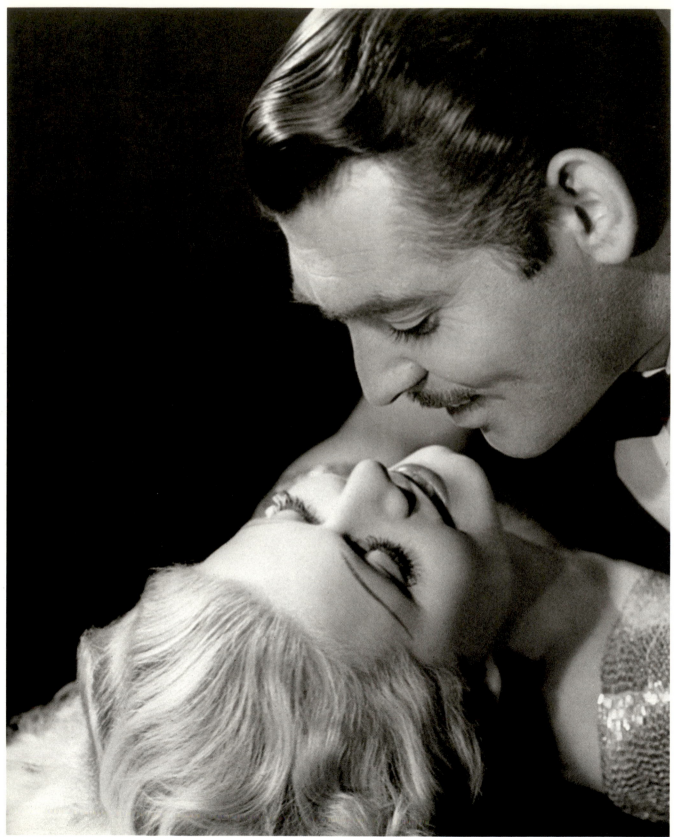

56

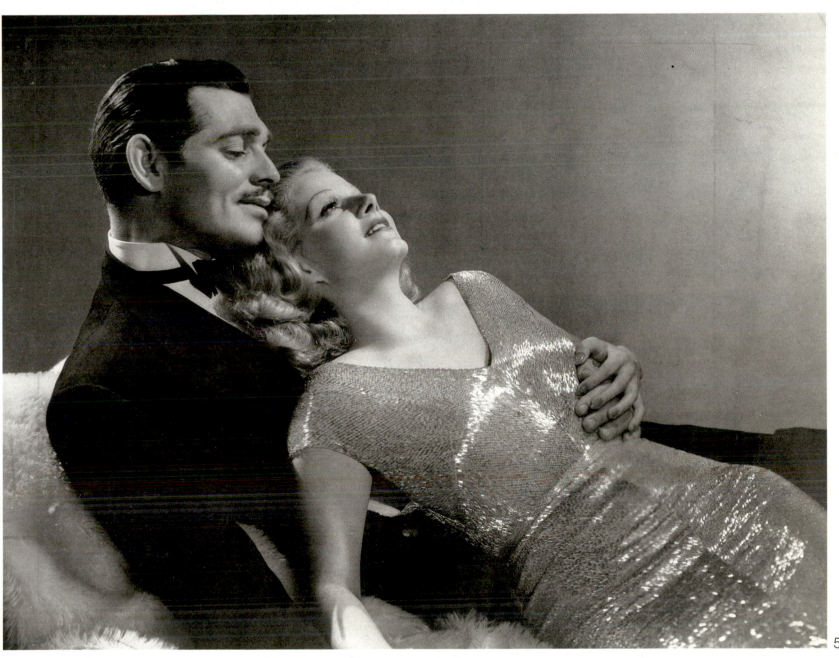

57

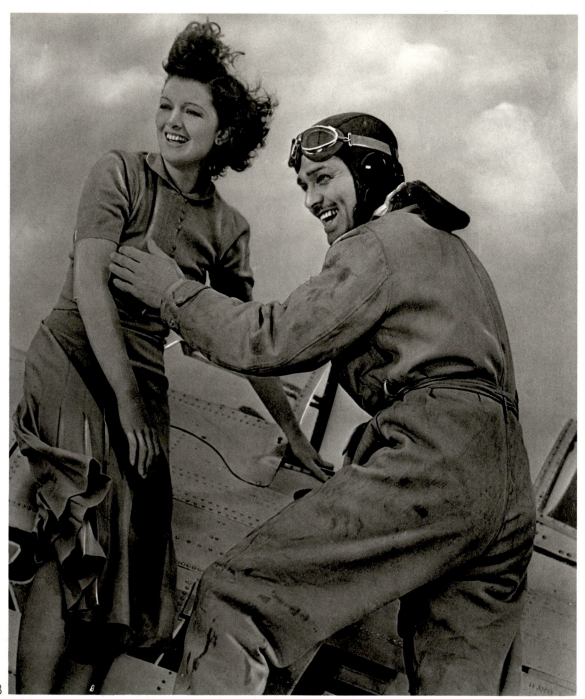

58

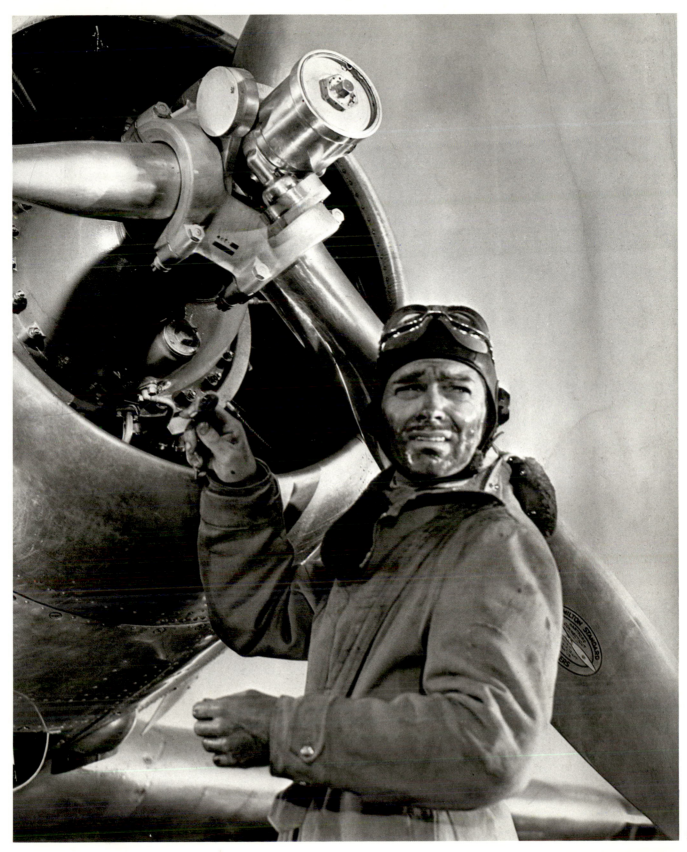

59

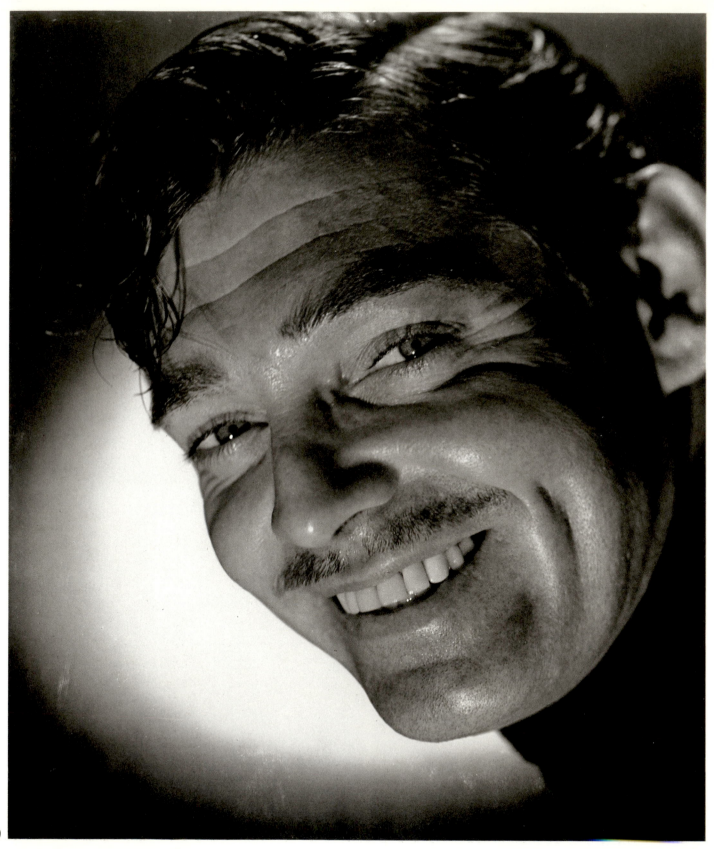

60

'. . . He radiated such charm and vitality that I began to see what people meant when they said a sort of magic happened when he was present. When he smiled his crooked smile he seemed much handsomer than he was on the screen.'

Jean Garceau
(Gable's personal secretary)

'There is no use trying to explain Clark Gable. He simply possesses, through the strange and fantastic medium of the camera, a dynamic and glittering force. Seen through the magic lens, he has that peculiar power to stimulate emotions in those who watch him, which is the one unfailing uniform characteristic of the few idols the screen has known.'

Adela Rogers St. John, 1932

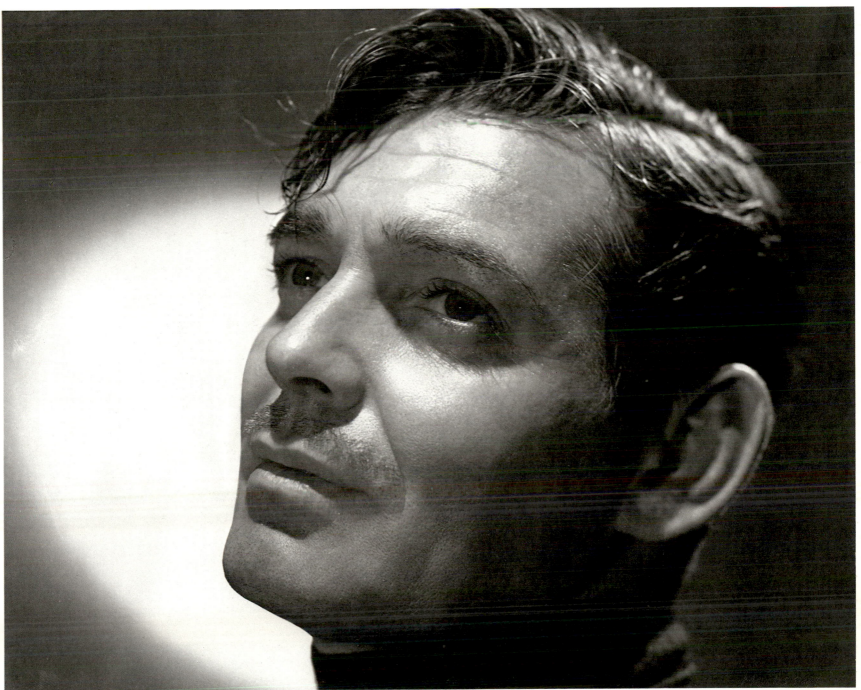

61

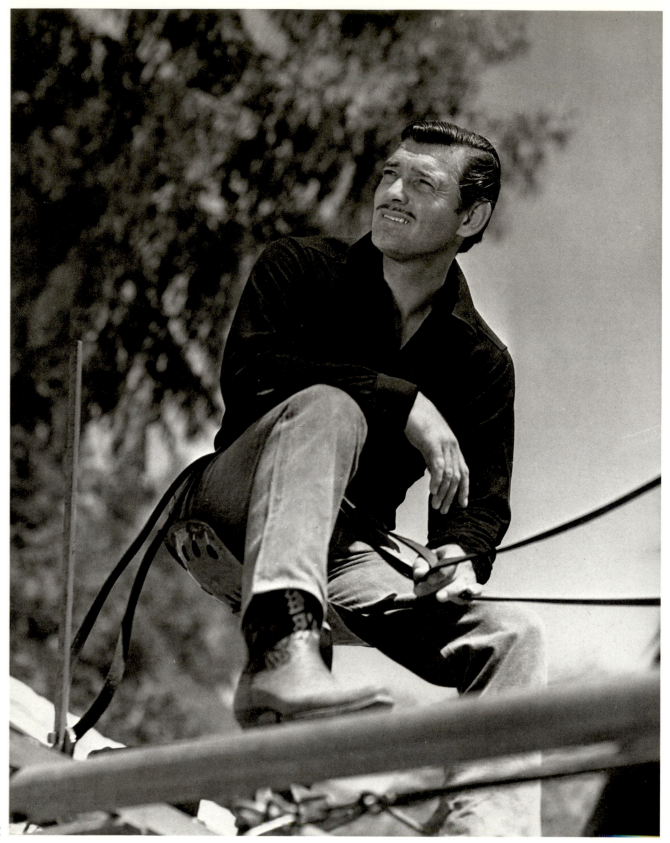

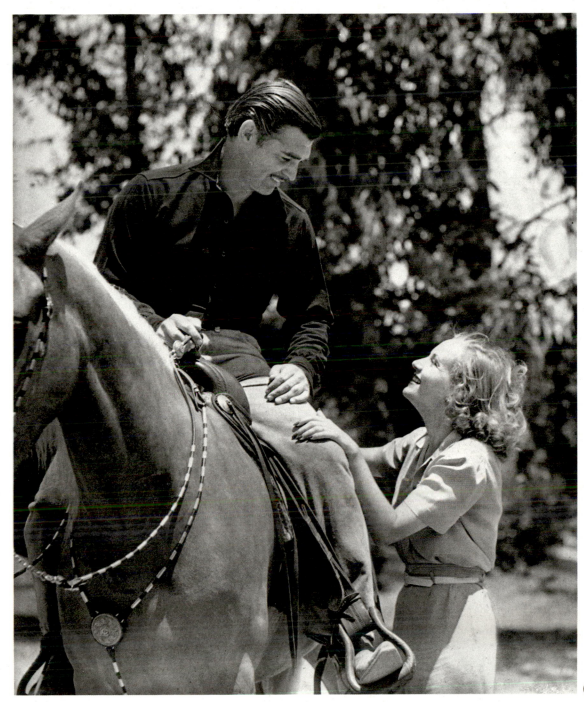

63

'Gable made villains popular. Instead of the audience wanting the good man to get the girl, they began wanting the bad man to get her.'

Norma Shearer

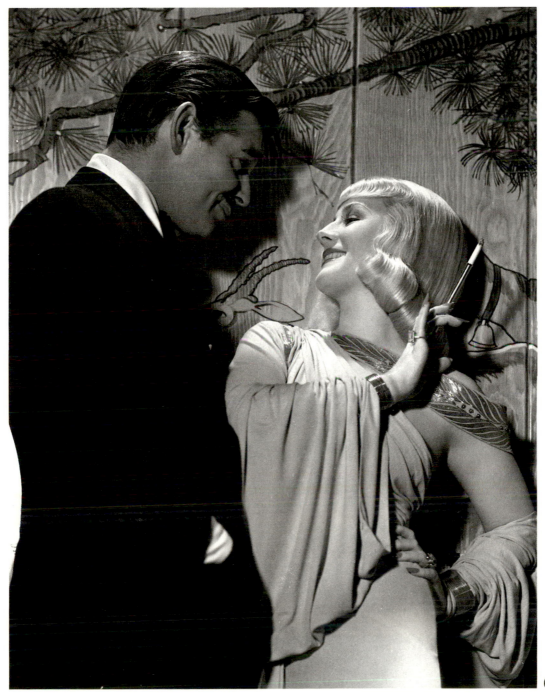

64

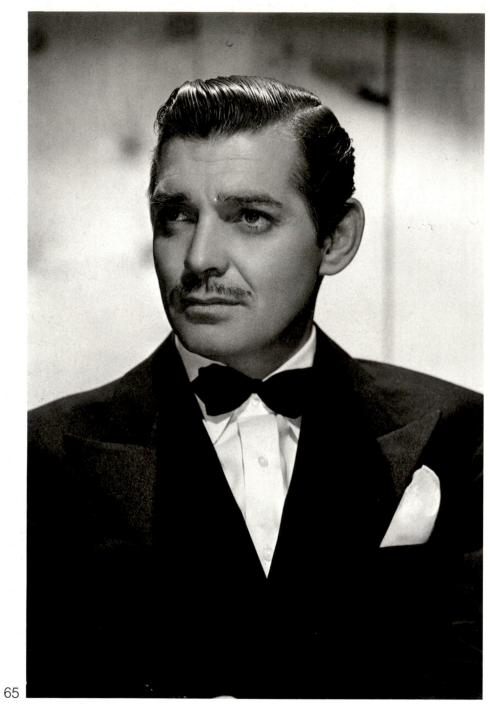

65

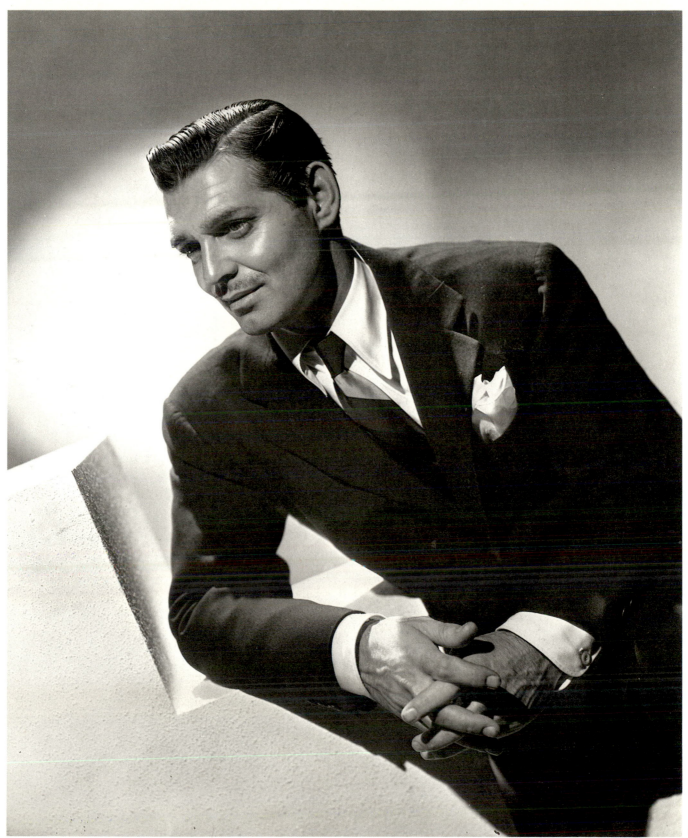

66

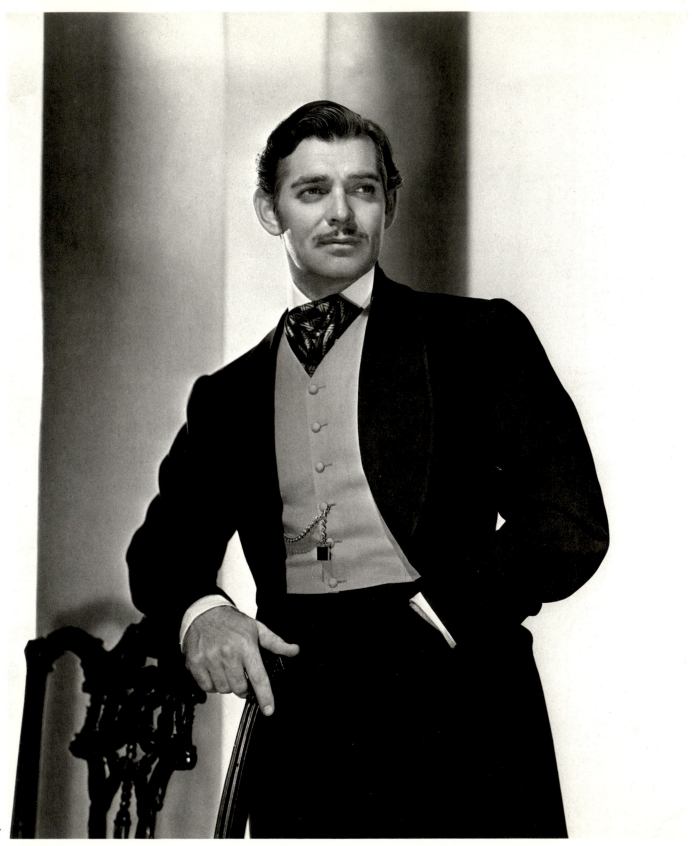

67

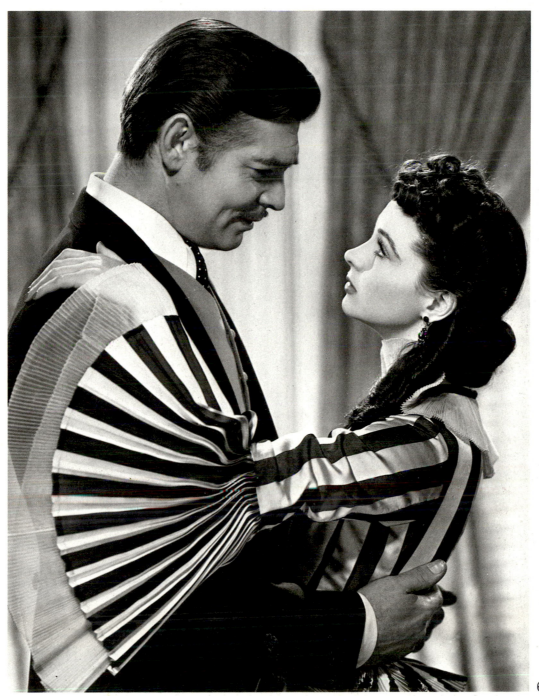

68

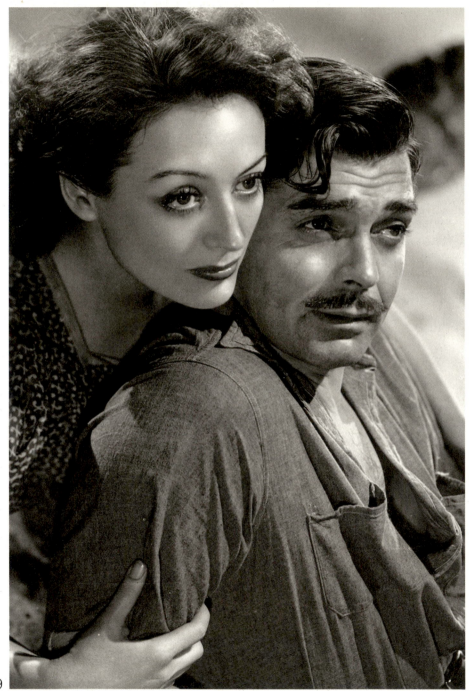

69

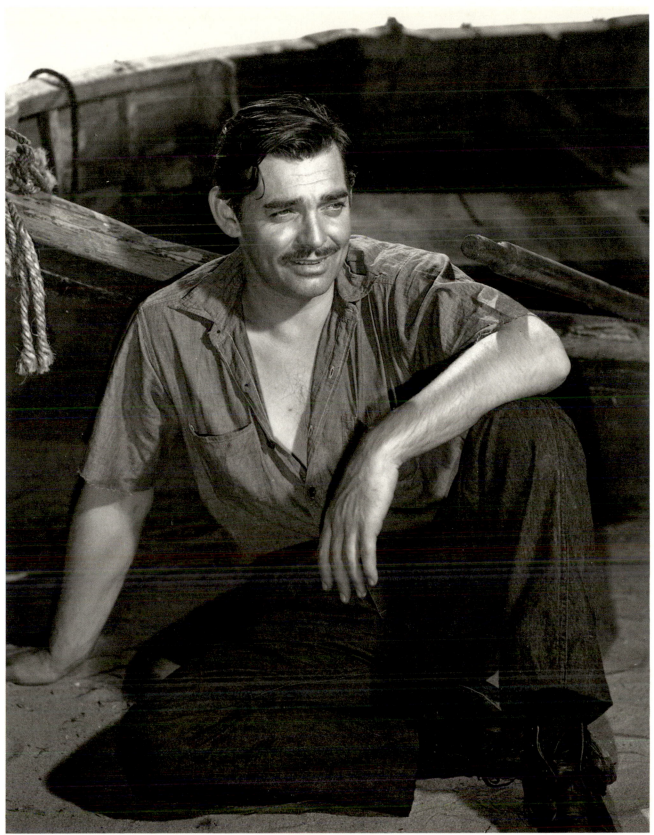

70

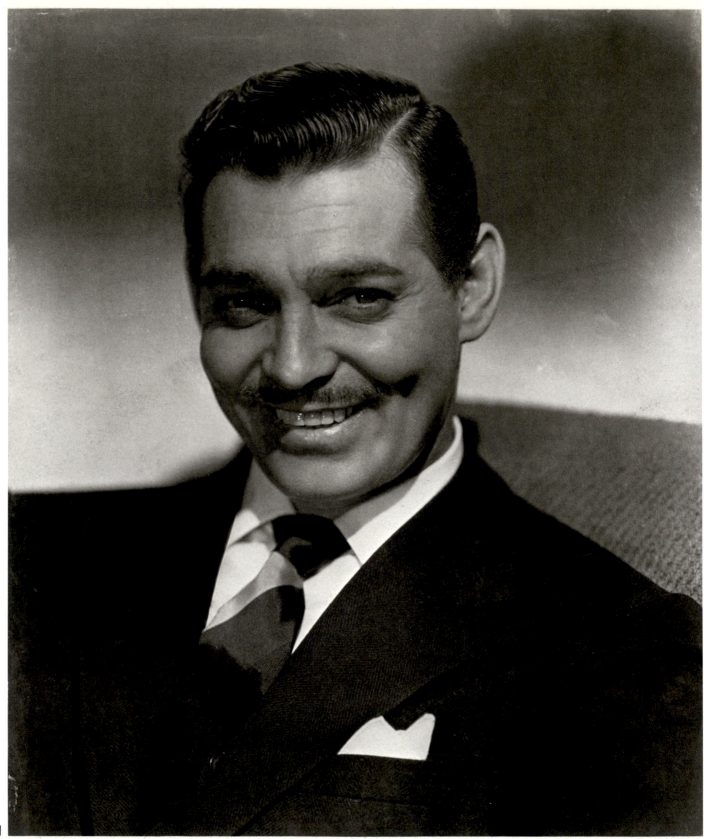

71

'I had never met Clark, and like every woman in the country, thought he was divine. I also jumped at the gay prospect of looking at him every day — and getting paid besides!'

Claudette Colbert,
after *It Happened One Night,* 1934

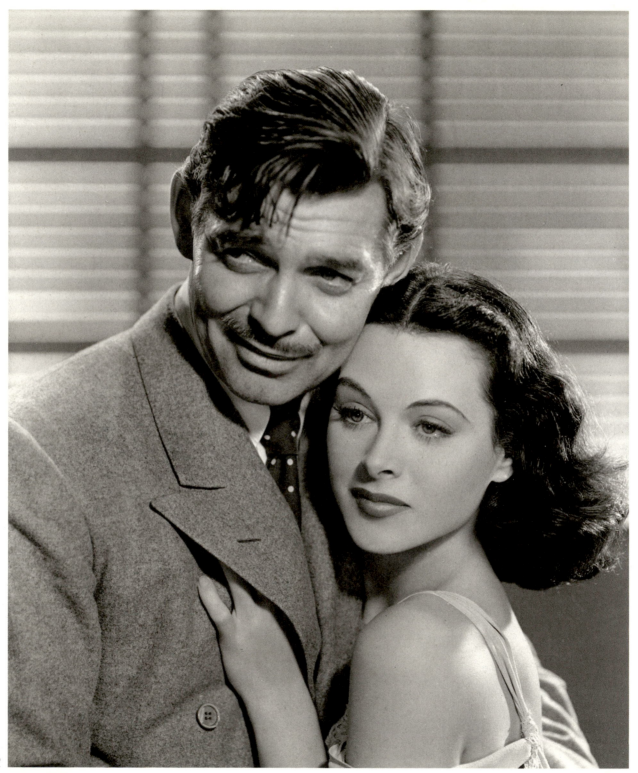

72

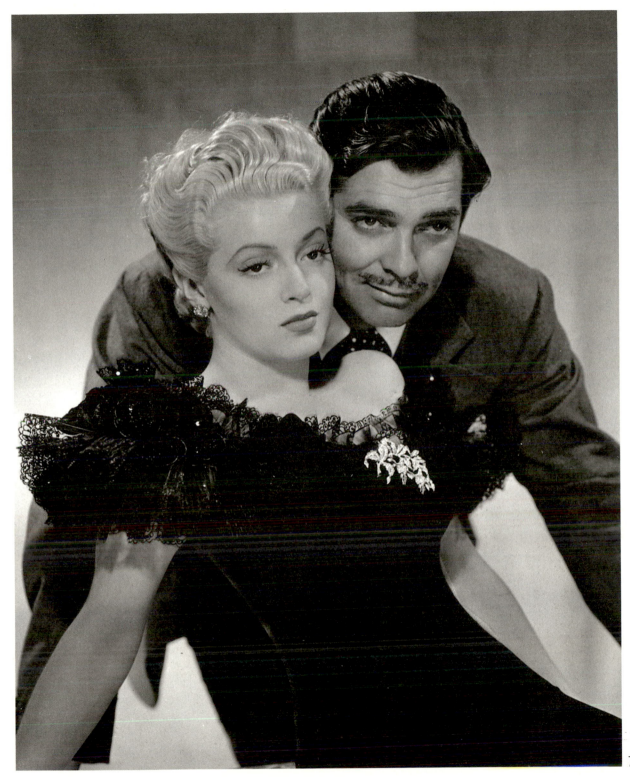

73

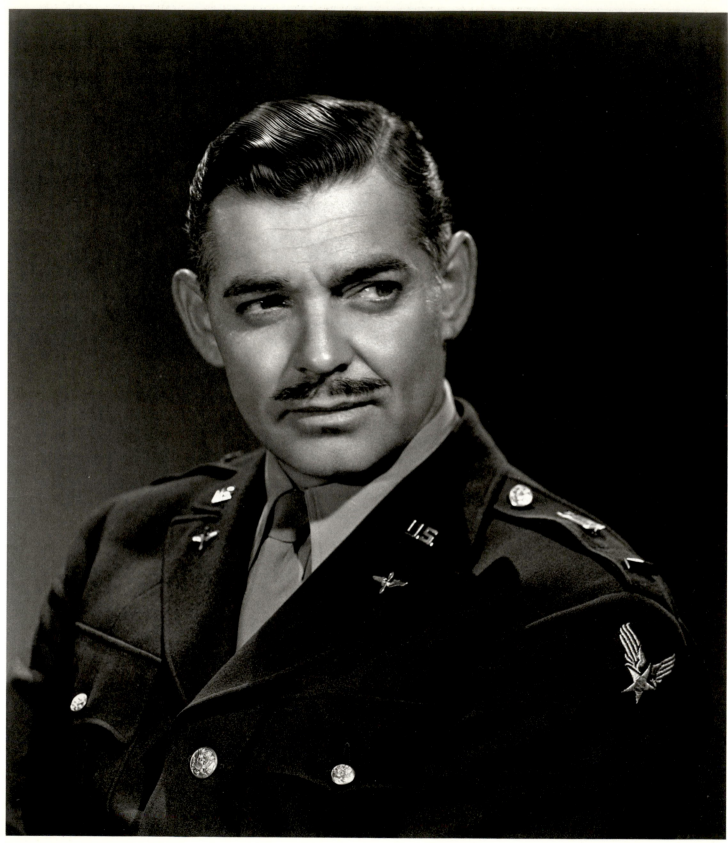

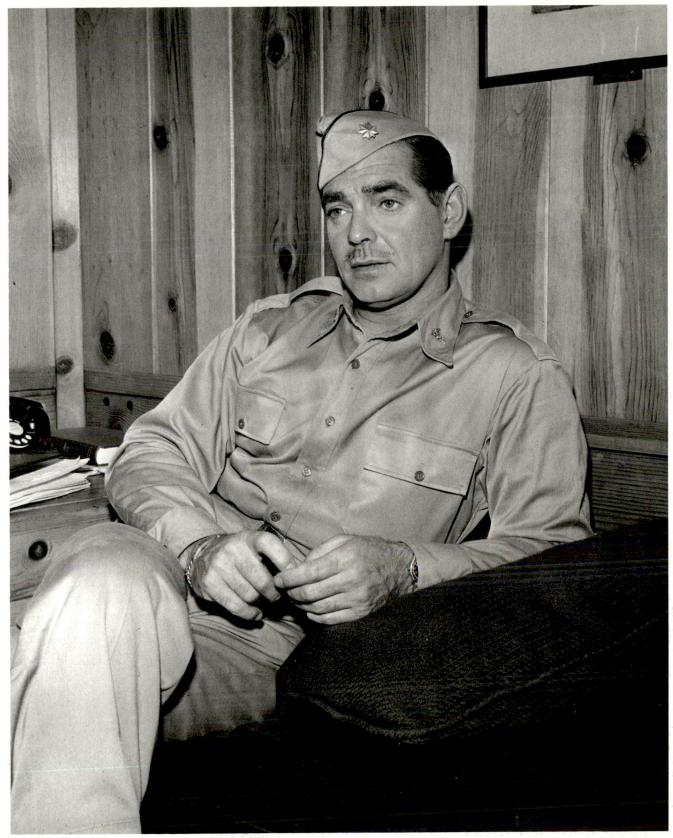

75

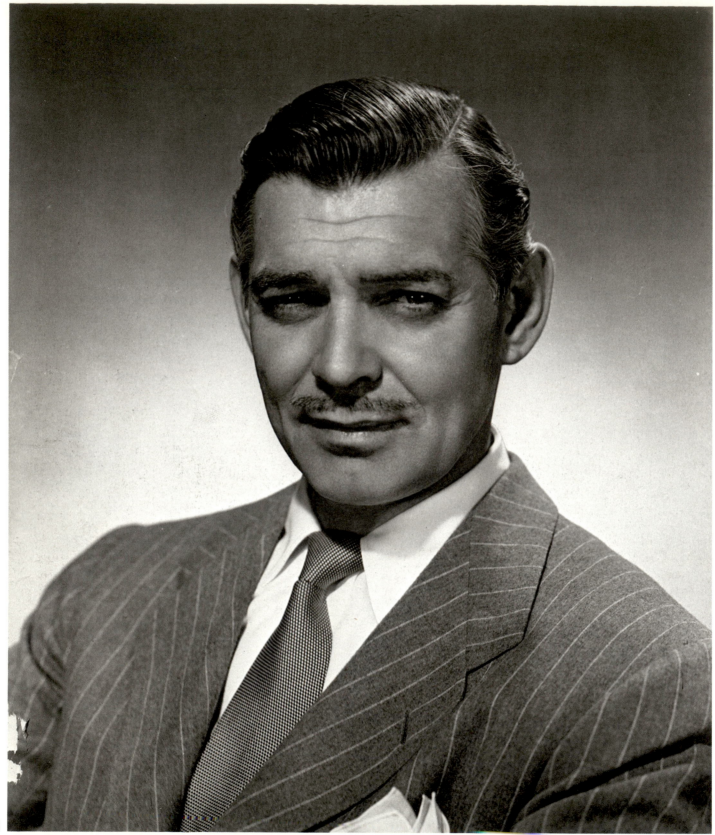

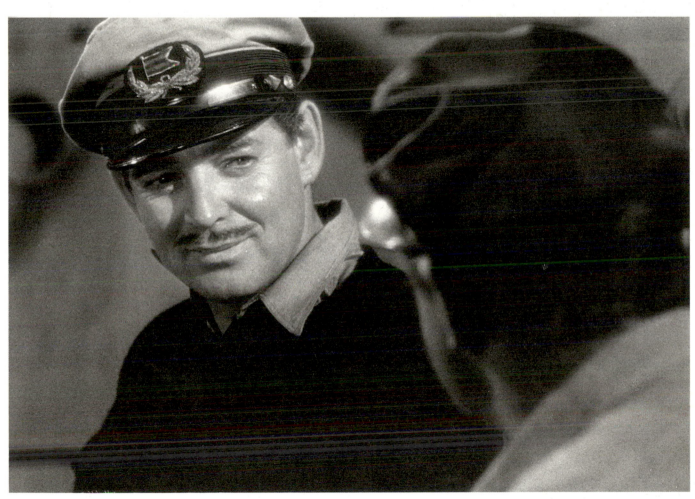

'I know I haven't fooled the public with these dinner-jacket parts I've been playing for the past year or more. What's more, I don't like to fool them even if I could. I'd like to get back to Gable the roughneck and forget Gable the gentleman. I guess what I really want more than anything else is a chance to be myself again, both on and off the screen.'

Clark Gable, 1934

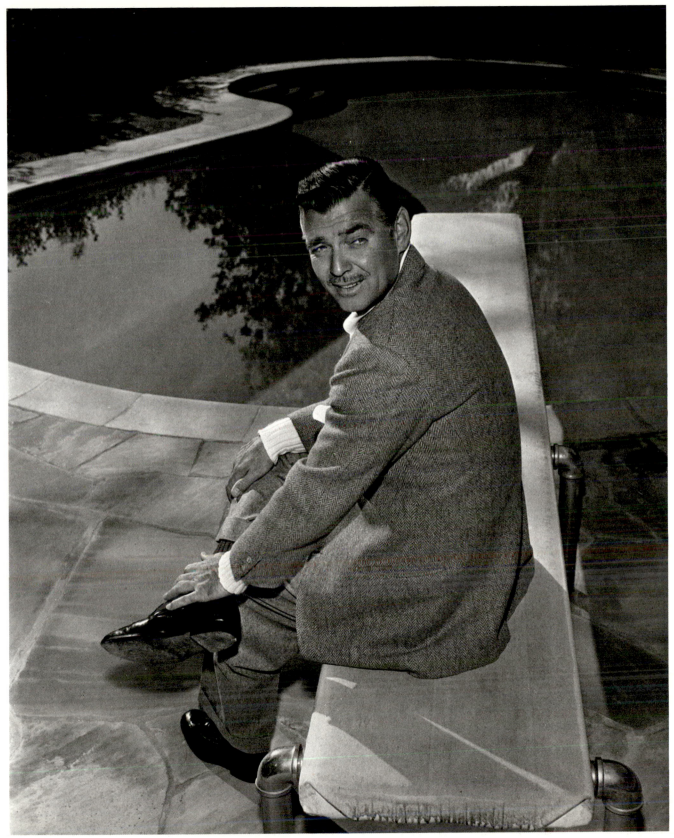

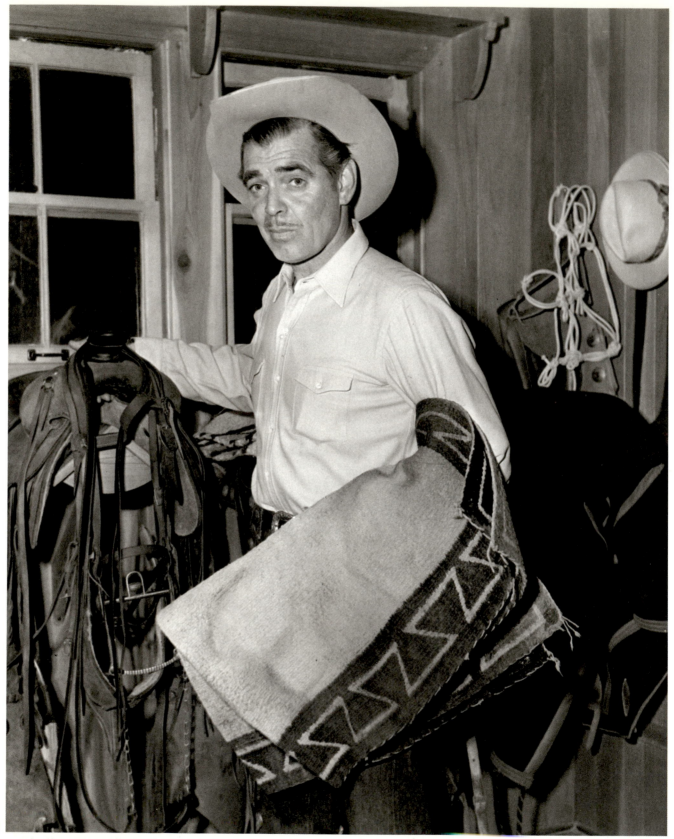

79

'When I was growing up, Clark Gable represented everything I idealised . . . and to find that ideal was all I ever dreamed of, plus so much more — more human, warmer! I am sorry he didn't always receive the recognition for his acting that he deserved, because he cared so very much.'

Marilyn Monroe

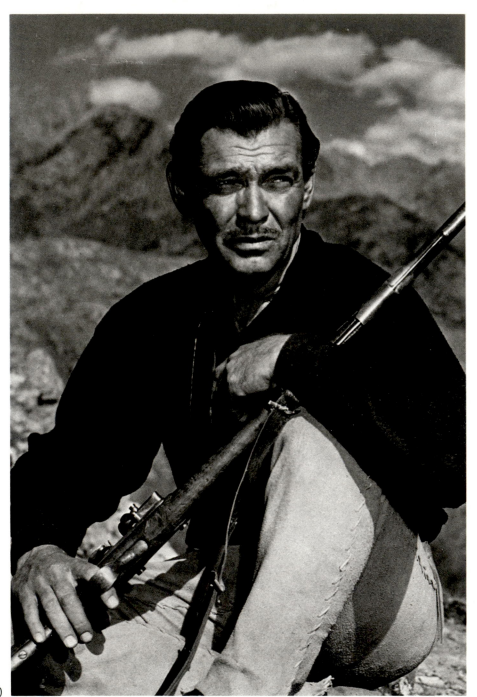

80

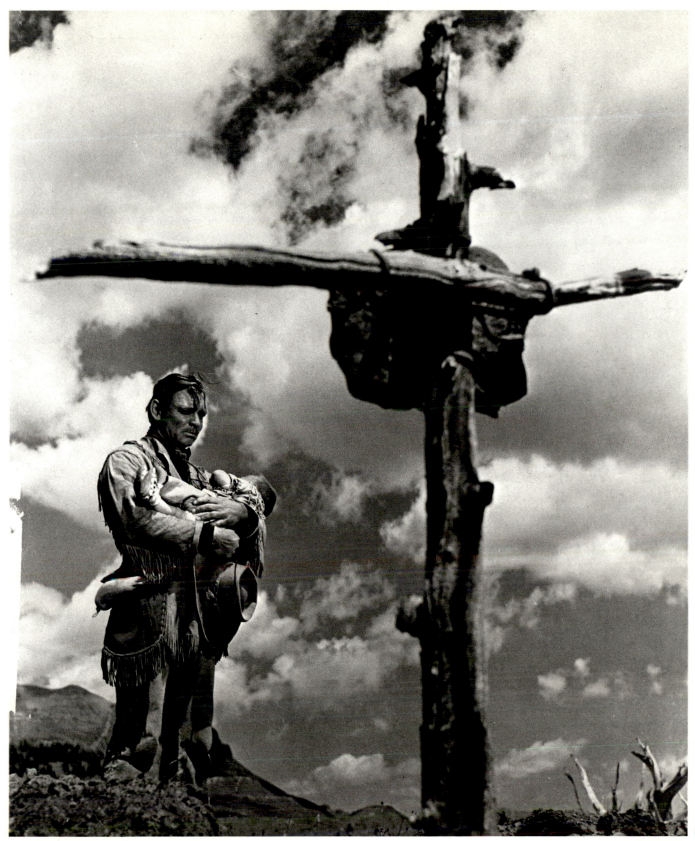

81

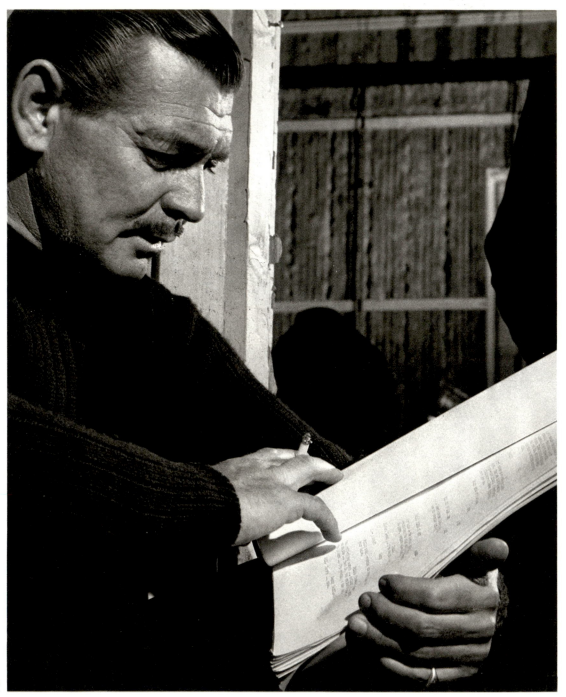

82

'I've never been able to connect stars with parts I write, but after meeting Gable I could see him as Gay Langland (*The Misfits*). He had the same sort of lyricism underneath, something one didn't usually think of, watching him. It was his secret charm – tough but responsive to feeling and ideals.'

Arthur Miller

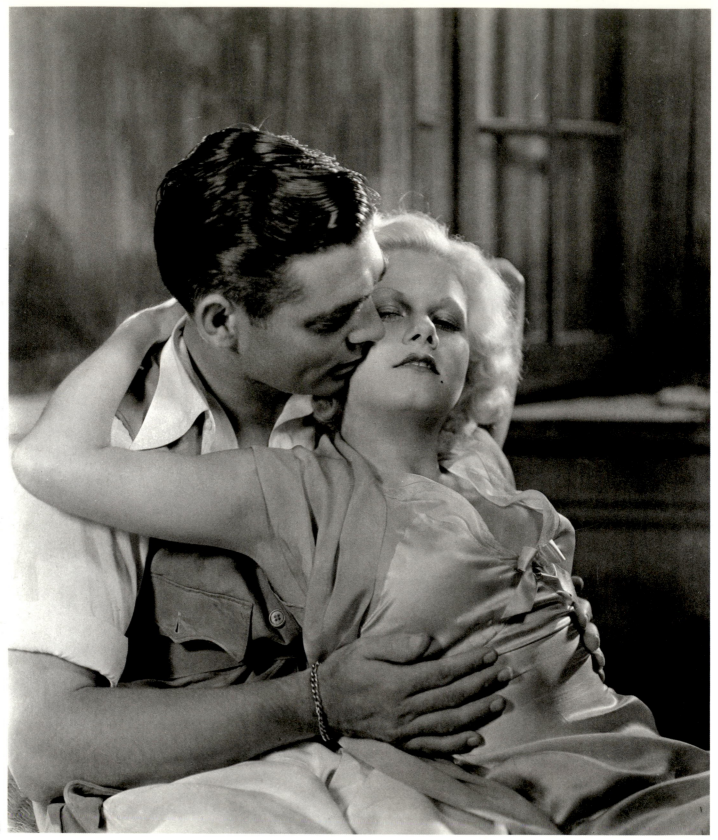

83

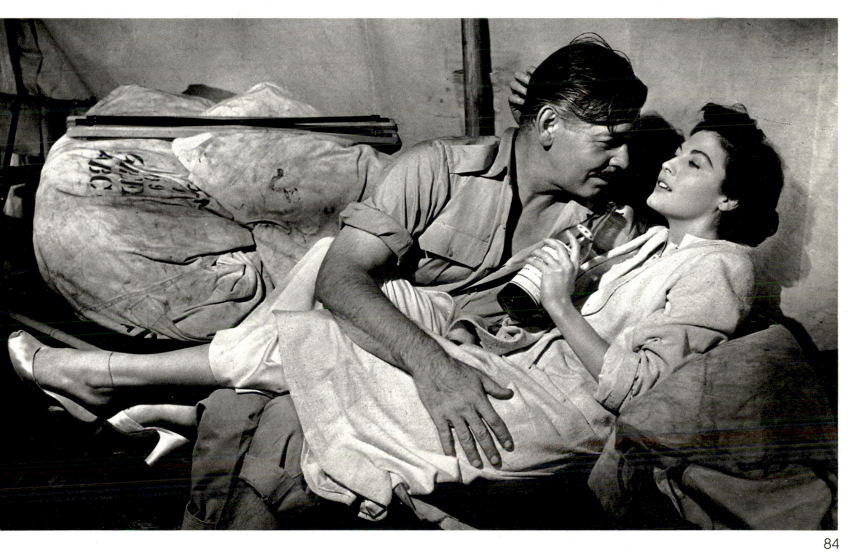

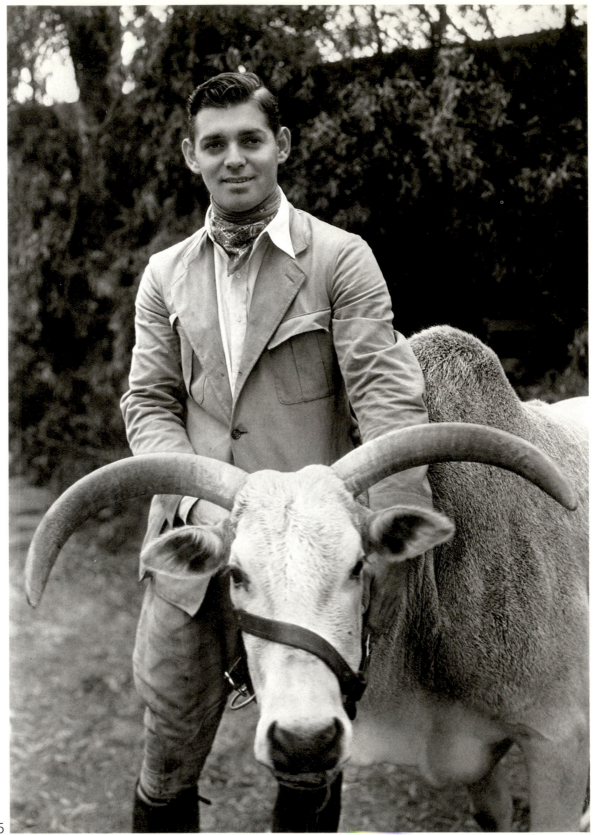

85

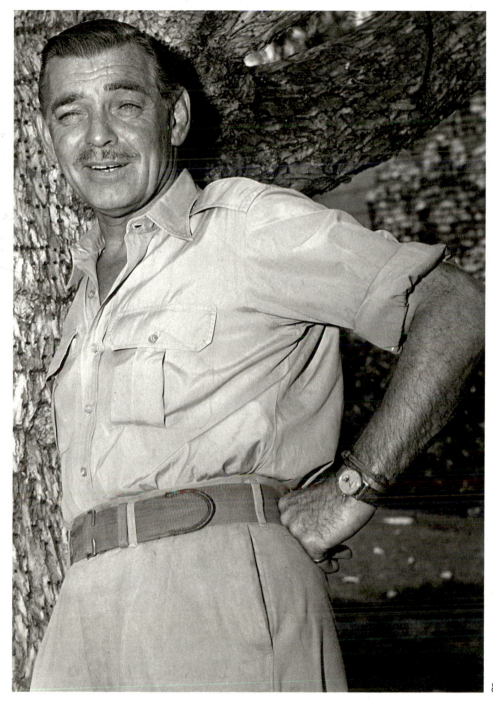

86

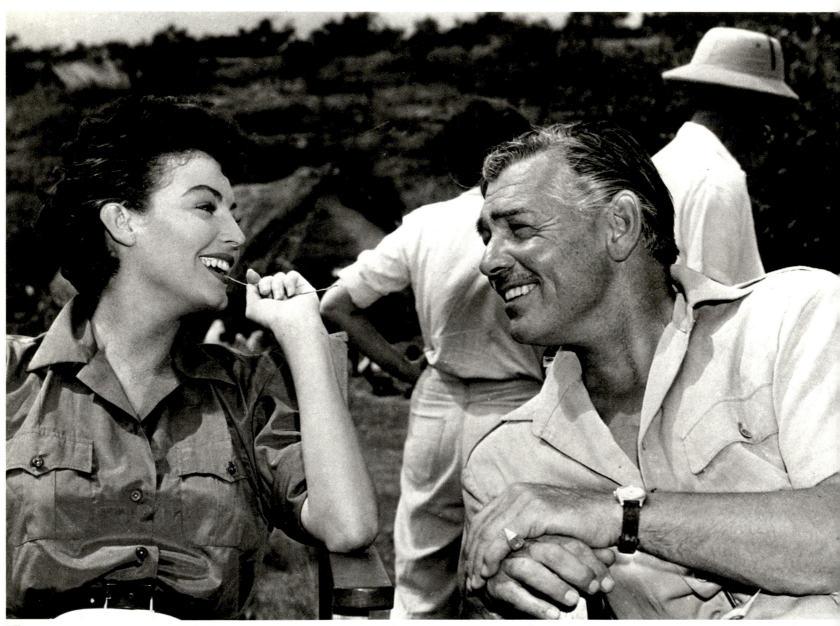

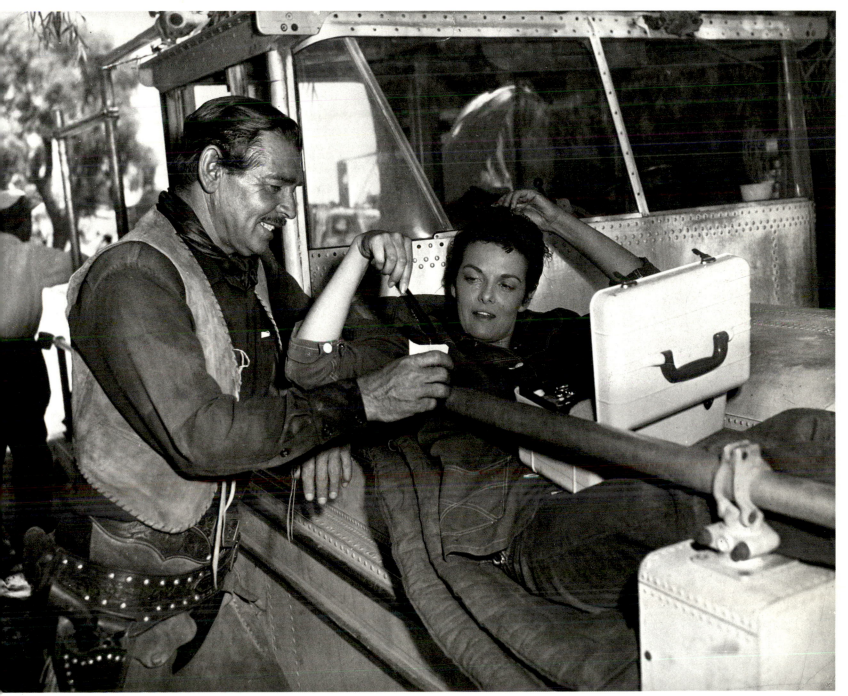

88

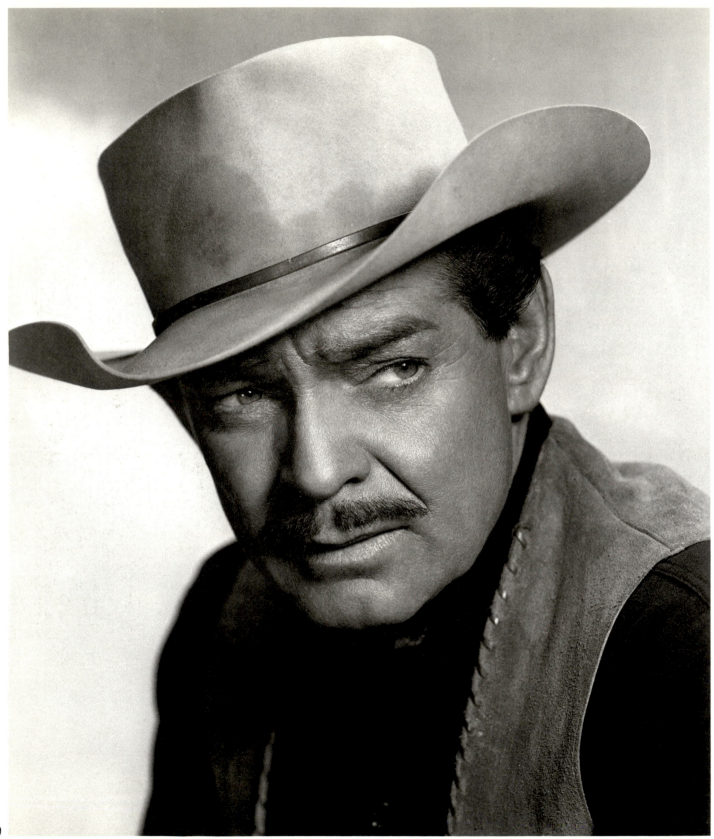

89

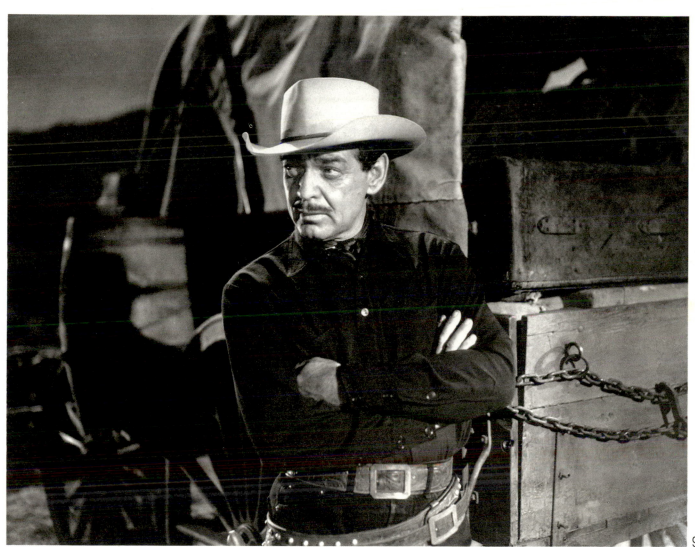

90

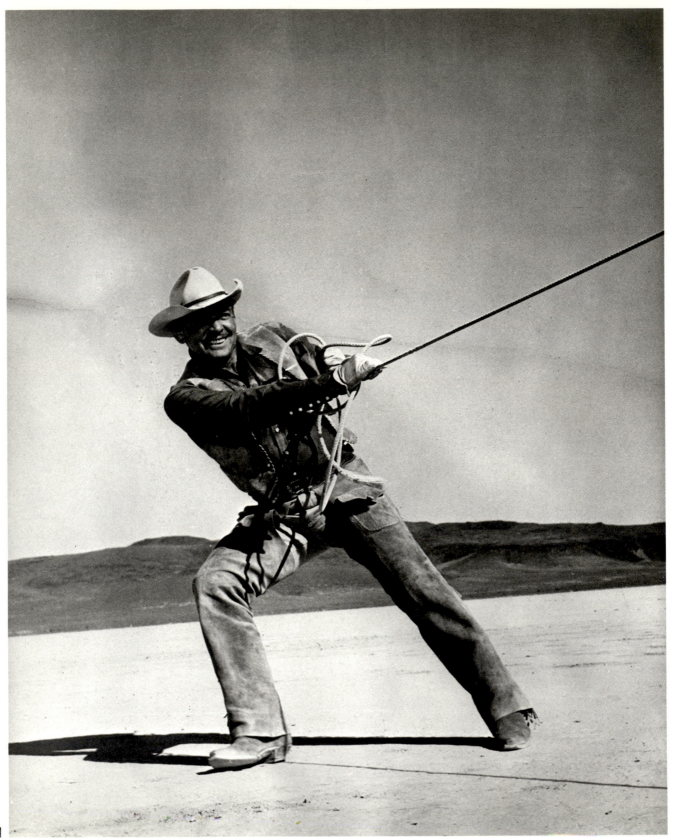

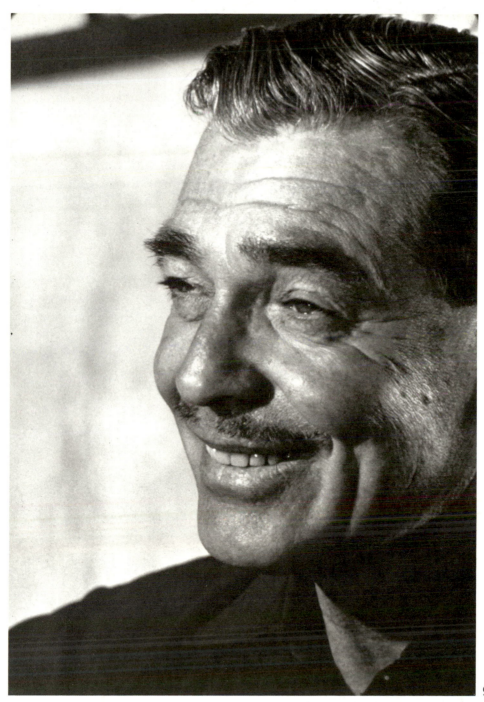

92

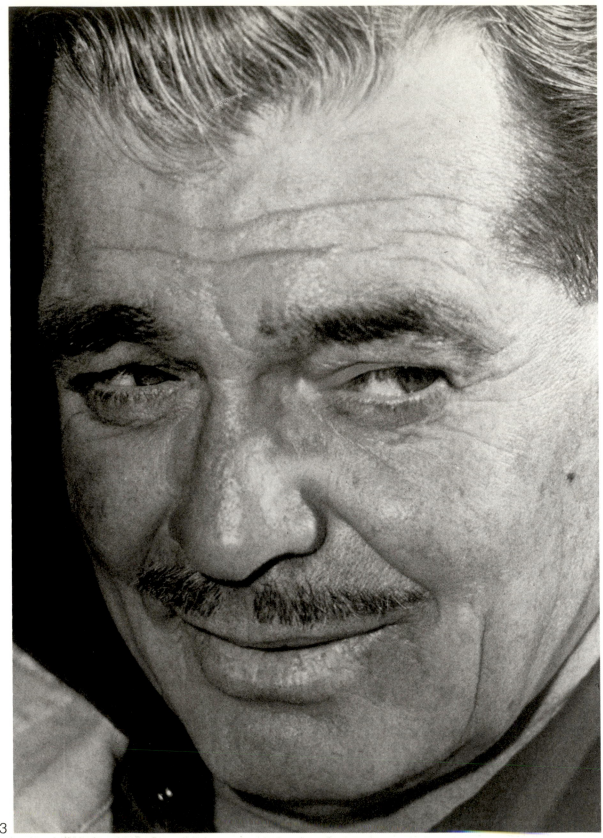

93

'Rare human qualities Mr. Gable possessed in an unusual degree: virility graced by humour, good nature adorned by comprehension, an easy manner unspoiled by pretensions. To these engaging traits he added professional integrity and personal sincerity not easily found in the competitive atmosphere of the screen.'

Editorial, *Los Angeles Times,*
on Gable's death

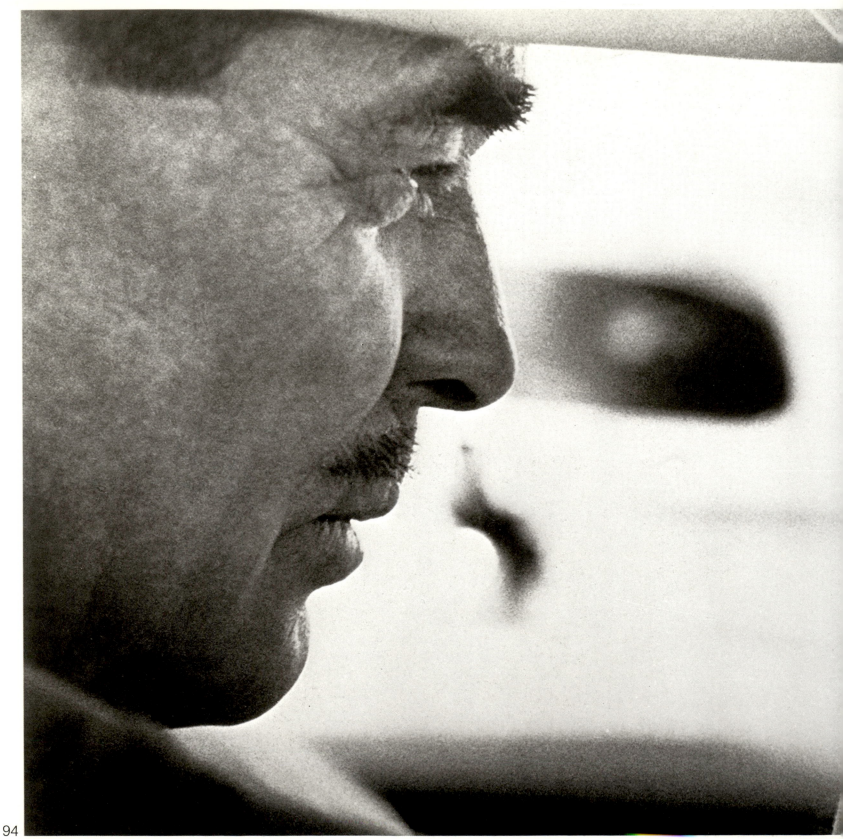

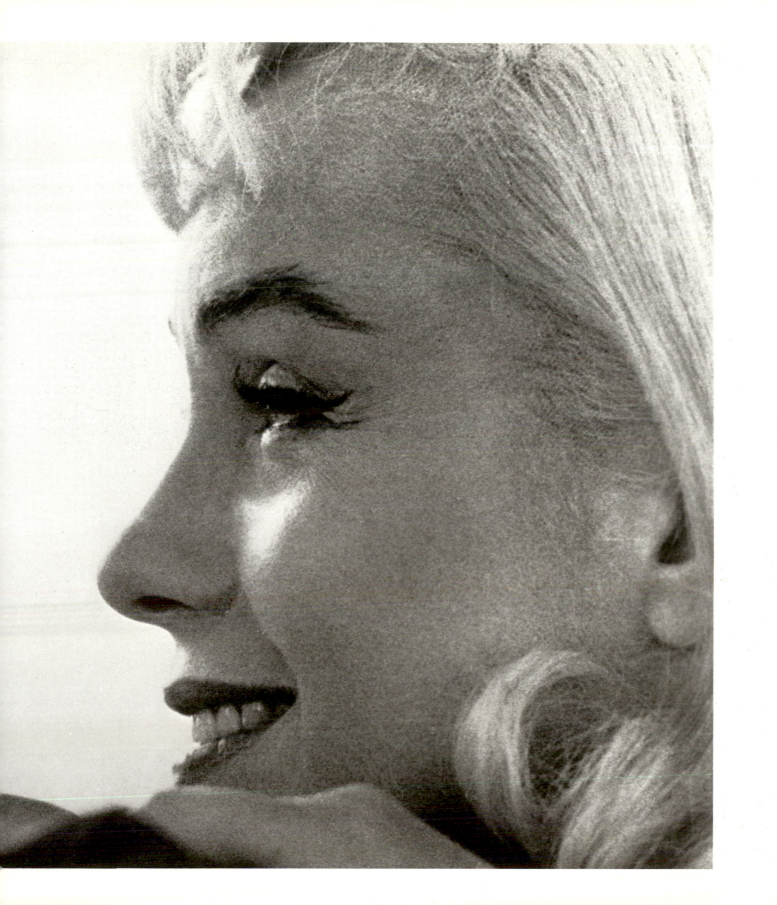

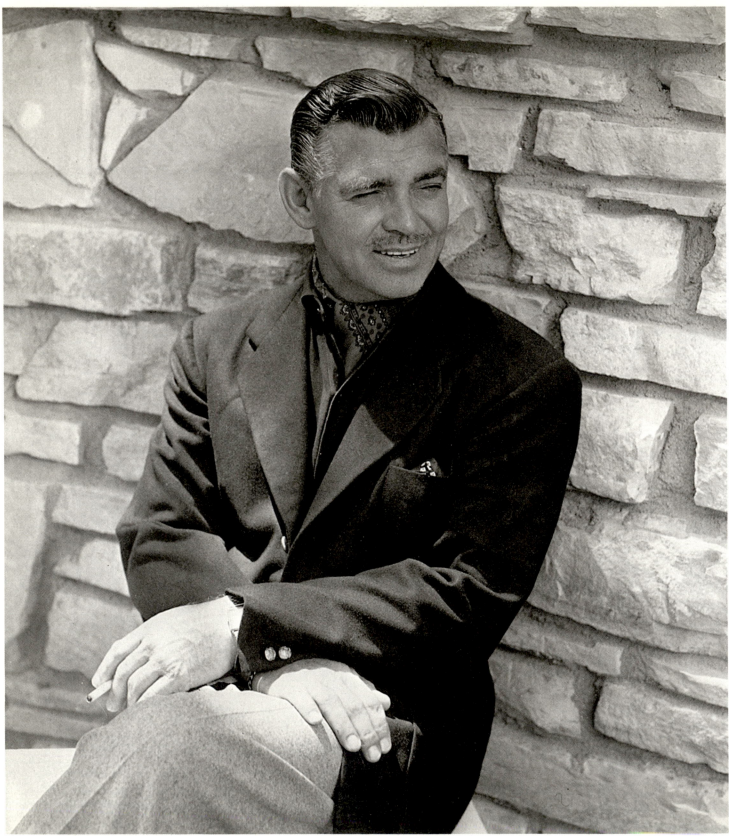

THE FILM STAR AS PHOTOGRAPHIC MODEL

Laszlo Willinger arrived in Hollywood in the summer of 1937 to work at M-G-M as the head of their portrait department. The stars, especially the great women stars like Joan Crawford, Norma Shearer, and Jean Harlow had been used to, and spoiled by, George Hurrell's brilliant portraits during that celebrated photographer's tenure at Metro. After he stormed out of there in 1932, they kept insisting on him despite the studio's other gallery photographers, like Clarence Sinclair Bull. Bull pleased Greta Garbo, who liked his quiet, reserved, discreetly professional approach to work, but the others did not all feel as secure or as disinterested in the necessary art of self-promotion and felt that only Hurrell could do them justice. This proved both extremely expensive to the studio as his free-lance price rose into the thousands but also deeply humiliating to the publicity department that had allowed him to get away. For the next five years they kept trying to find a photographer whose work would please their demanding stable of stars, and who would also be under contract to them.

Part of the problem was solved when Jean Harlow liked the work of one young local photographer, Ted Allan, and he became her photographer for the last few years of her brief life. But it was with the advent of the Austro-Hungarian photographer Laszlo Willinger that the others capitulated. Norma Shearer adored what he did for her, so did Crawford, and the less demanding but equally professional Myrna Loy. The great male stars under contract, Clark Gable, Spencer Tracy, Nelson Eddy, Robert Taylor, Fred Astaire . . . were somewhat less fussy, or professed to be, but they too relaxed and opened up with Willinger. Later on, when such stars as Hedy Lamarr, Louise Rainer, Greer Garson and Vivien Leigh, as well as such starlets groomed for stardom like Lana Turner, Lucille Ball and others joined, Laszlo did some of their most memorable sessions.

His photographs gave them an aura of allure coupled with intelligence, and, a charming surprising quality of modesty about these otherwise remote creatures: as if they too realized that there was a world out there besides the high paid one of make-believe they inhabited, and in their bearing before his camera they seemed to convey that awareness without losing their attractive larger than life quality: Crawford seemed to become reflective, Norma Shearer had a touch of spring about her; Myrna Loy had a living-room smile and the bedroom in her eyes was now a special glint for just the right man. Willinger's Vivien Leigh portraits for *Waterloo Bridge* and *Gone With the Wind* captured better than any photographs of her before or after, the moment when stardom hits, before it pales, and when forever after, on seeing these portraits he took of her, one can see and say, that is why Vivien Leigh was a sensation. There is a secret and a difference, a surprise and a bold defiance of what tomorrow might bring. No wonder that the unwilling star asked Laszlo to come to San Francisco where she was playing Juliet to Olivier's Romeo and ask him to take their special portraits.

But Laszlo's success was not just in capturing the women stars. In fact, some of his finest work is of men and possibly the best of all are his portraits of the decade's most lionized, idolized star, Clark Gable. Every star has that moment when everything he/she was going to be meets up and forever defines his/her appeal. The portraits Laszlo took of Gable capture both that moment and that appeal. These portraits show Gable as a man in the prime of his life and on top of the world. There is still a touch of the cruelly handsome and slightly dangerous Lothario – in which guise Gable first cracked across the screen (after discouraging years of hanging around one should add) when he co-starred as a night-club owning gangster in the Joan Crawford film, *Dance Fools Dance* and as the man who smacked ladylike Norma Shearer around in *A Free Soul*. But in these Willinger sessions, the brutish caveman is now concentrated in an engaging twinkle in the eyes as well as by that forever roguish smile and the slight sense one gets of tension in the brows above the eye. A lot had happened since those two early 1930/31 films.

Initially, Gable's brute male approach had helped revolutionise America's idea of the romantic lover. With the advent of actors like Gable and Cagney gone were the discreet, gentlemanly lovers of silent films. Everything about Gable was direct, straight on, even his eyes and his crooked clean shaven smile were two fisted. He was a man who would not be buried by the depression – his looks were not for dreaming, or so one would believe from the roughing up he gave his leading ladies as easily as he could punch his way out of a gang of men.

By 1937 and Willinger, his brand of appeal had been broadened, refined, made more accessible so that when the gangster era was over, he would not fall by the wayside the way others do when the tide of fashion turns. Not that there was any need to worry. Audiences liked to see him in anything whether comedy, drama, romantic soap-operas, adventure . . . the lot.

Willinger arrived at Metro at the precise moment when the definitive Gable image clicked in. The photos that came out of their sessions in the gallery are as definitive in their way of who Gable was, what he meant, and why he should have lasted so long and survived so many changes, as in their way, Hurrell's surrealistic portraits of Jean Harlow or Bachrach's extravagant portraits of the coltish Kate Hepburn, and all the other great, timeless sessions to come out of the 50 years of Hollywood's role in providing us with role models. Willinger brings us this Gable, cocky but nice, self-assured but endearing. Gable is playing with the camera, he is putting on that endearing look; he is very confident with his facial expressions; all the more surprising since at the outset of his career, one of his major drawbacks when looking for work was the fact that his ears were not only large but stood out and would have to be taped back, and he knew, even if his public didn't, that his gleaming white teeth were false. Here is a man who doesn't feel his appeal rests on his appearance and that is what makes his appearance so appealing. From these Willinger portraits, the first ones taken three years before he was signed to play Rhett in *Gone With The Wind*, it become apparent why his casting was a foregone conclusion, why in fact the book's author, Margaret Mitchell, confided that when she was writing the book, she had Gable in mind as the prototype for her fictional hero.

These portraits belong to Gable's best work. This is how we remember him and how he remained for the rest of his life, older, wiser but still that same cocky, endearing Gable – a man who had learned to live with being a legend.

JOHN KOBAL

ON PHOTOGRAPHING CLARK GABLE

Gable had something extremely rare, he looked good from any angle. Most people have a good and bad side, best from one angle only. He could be photographed under any lighting conditions, any camera angle. There was another, probably more important factor. He was the least self-conscious person in front of the camera. Myrna Loy was like Gable in this respect. She seemed to be at ease with herself and saw posing for stills as another part of her profession, which she took seriously. As I said in the past, professionals can smell each other and are comfortable with each other and she certainly respected me as a fellow professional. And then, on the other end of the scale, there was Marilyn Monroe whose whole life revolved around the camera. She only came to life when she saw that glass eye pointed at her. Basically, she was a dilettante who always feared that she might be found out. But the camera was safe; it avoided the need of her dealing with real people on a one-to-one basis. As she told me once when I marvelled at her ability to go in a fraction of a second from next to nothing to a lifelike imitation of sparkling vivacity only to drop into dull mediocrity after she heard the click of the camera, 'This is like being screwed by a hundred guys and you can't get pregnant!' Well, Gable simply took it for granted that the man behind the camera was as professional as he was and that both worked for the same purpose, to make him look as appealing as possible.

Most stars, even men, insisted on seeing proofs of all photos taken and they made their own selection of what they permitted to be published. They interfered with the lighting, even the backgrounds, and were deeply concerned with what should be retouched. They even insisted that all original negatives rejected by them be destroyed. Joan Crawford and Norma Shearer to mention two who had that privilege and who exercised it and, of all people, Nelson Eddy. When casting began for *Gone With The Wind*, Gable showed up at my studio in a Confederate uniform, with a sideburn and a moustache and said, 'I want you to shoot some pictures of me in this get-up.' Rather intrigued, I asked him why he wanted these pictures and without smiling he said, 'Don't you see, I AM Rhett Butler.' Those negs were destroyed by our common decision before anyone else ever saw them . . . Gable was sure enough of himself never to bother with such details.

I once talked to him about his easygoing attitude and he said, 'I am getting paid to be in front of the camera and you are getting paid to be behind it and the bosses seem to be satisfied with both of us, so why worry?' He liked his pictures and said so, but it was no great thing for him, or for that matter, for me. Of course, we talked while I was shooting, but mostly it was chit-chat. He was not interested in the mechanics of photography. He simply assumed that I knew my business. He never asked me to photograph his wife, nor did he, to my knowledge, ever ask for any special prints and certainly not to give as gifts to anybody. He was not vain or so presumptuous as to give pictures of himself as gifts. Gable had two distinctly different personalities. When he appeared at official functions, he was the quintessential movie star; he could make an entrance into a room worthy of a Barrymore. He was adept at talking to the press by making the least important cub reporter feel as though he had just got the scoop of the century. To him this was part of the performance for which he was paid. And then there was the other Gable. He was most comfortable away from Hollywood, fishing, hunting . . . mostly with people who had never been in a gossip column. He was given to corny practical jokes. Once, when he was married to Carole Lombard, he gave her as a birthday gift a big ham, adorned with a pink bow. Another time he bought an old rusty jallopy and, without changing its exterior, put a high-performance motor in it just to enjoy the thrill of taking off at 60 miles from a standing start to the amazement of all other drivers on the road. And after work he was often seen sitting around a less than elegant bar across the street from the studio with his cronies . . . electricians, grips, carpenters . . . having a wonderful time being just one of the boys.

He was a man who got what he wanted, never raising his voice and never making enemies . . . indeed a rare exception in Hollywood – then and now – where posturing and self-congratulation are thought to be essential tools of the trade.

When I had to photograph Gable with someone else, for example, when we had to do publicity photographs of the stars which could be used for poster art, Gable didn't demand any prerogative. When I shot him and Joan Crawford for *Strange Cargo* Crawford had to be lighted carefully, Gable got the leak light from the spot on her. At the time I was told they had a short-lived affair, but I have no first-hand knowledge. It certainly wasn't apparent in the way they worked. From what his occasional girls rather indiscreetly conveyed to one and all, he was no great shakes in bed and I am convinced that all Crawford needed for sexual rapture was a mirror. It wasn't lighting he was worried about, just a professional attitude when it came to work. When I was doing the two shots of him with Norma Shearer for *Idiot's Delight* I had the distinct feeling that Gable did not particularly care for her, especially because she kept him (and everybody else) waiting for hours until she made her regal entry on the set and then . . . did not know her lines. He became visibly annoyed when she dithered with her make-up, her hair, her dress etc. when he had been ready for an hour.

There was no difference in my approach to shooting in Hollywood, Paris, Berlin or Vienna. Hollywood was easier for me because the crews were immeasurably more competent. And, of course, sets were built especially according to my instructions, something unheard of in Europe. Everything was made easy In Hollywood . . . as long as the results were good.

As for cameras, lights etc that we used at MGM when I first got there: the standard camera was an 8 × 10 view camera with 12 to 15 inch lenses. Even the photographers on the set used this unwieldy monster. There was no candid camera used in the studios other than a heavy 5 × 7 Graflex which sounded like a pistol shot when it took the exposure. Not until *Life* and *Look* sent their photographers with the 35 mm cameras was there any change . . . and that came very slowly. On the set the photographer, using the lighting of the motion picture first, the camera man rushed into the set with his big camera and recreated a particular moment of the scene by posing the actors. Directors hated them; it took valuable time from their shooting.

One reason for using large format film was that it could be retouched; everything was retouched before the prints were made. Also, the hundreds of prints sent out every day were contact prints . . . the same size as the negative. This made it possible to make prints in a much quicker progression than by putting the negs into the enlarger and blowing them up to 8 × 10.

While I also used 8 × 10 film, I insisted that I make master prints myself through an enlarger. This gave me the luxury of composing as I wanted and to intensify or reduce certain portions of the image according to my idea of what the finished product should look like. Then a dupe neg was made from my master print and that was then used to make contact prints on which my corrections were incorporated . . . permanently.

For lights I used primary spotlights. They are lights with lenses which allowed me literally to paint with light, putting emphasis on certain areas, pinpointing what I considered the most flattering or important area of the composition while leaving unimportant areas in the shade. This was even more dramatic through my making the master print.

Today's system of throwing an overall flat light over everything, washing out all shadows and shooting with motorized cameras and hoping that out of a hundred frames one might get one good one is the exact opposite of what I did. I tried to make a photograph as dramatic as possible by lighting dramatically. That is impossible with today's lighting. Now the photographer is totally dependent on the absolute perfection of his model. Today the model is far more important than the photographer; this, no doubt is the reason that models have become stars in their own right. And quite rightly so. Today's photographer is an observer rather than a creator. He photographs what there is; I photographed what there ought to be. Of course, Clark Gable brought a lot of what there ought to be with him.

LASZLO WILLINGER

THE PHOTOGRAPHS

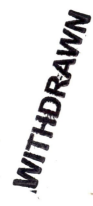

Phrase by Phrase

Pronunciation and Listening in American English

MARSHA CHAN
Mission College

PRENTICE HALL REGENTS

Library of Congress Cataloging-in-Publication Data

Chan, Marsha J., (date)
  Phrase by phrase.

  1. English language—Text-books for foreign
speakers. 2. English language—United States—
Pronunciation. 3. Listening. I. Title.
PE1128.C49 1987   428.3'4   86-25184
ISBN 0-13-665852-0

Editorial/production supervision and interior design:
  Ann L. Mohan, WordCrafters Editorial Services, Inc.
Cover design: Lundgren Graphics, Ltd.
Cover illustration: Ellen Joy Sasaki
Manufacturing buyer: Margaret Rizzi
Illustrator: Ellen Joy Sasaki

Material from "Three Days to See," by Helen Keller, is reprinted with kind
permission from American Foundation for the Blind and is © 1980 by American
Foundation for the Blind, 15 West 16th Street, New York, NY 10011.

Printed in the United States of America

 20 19 18 17 16 15

ISBN 0-13-665852-0

Contents

3   WHAT'S FOR DINNER?   21

4   JOHN THORNTON'S LOVE FOR BUCK   33

5   CLEANING UP THE BACKYARD   43

6 A SUNDAY OUTING 53

7 THE OAK AND THE REED 65

8 KOKO'S KITTEN 75

15   BABY BOOMERS: THE BIG BULGE   151

16   THE GIFT OF SIGHT   163

Introduction

Phrase by Phrase: Pronunciation and Listening in American English is a text-tape program designed for learners of English who wish to make their speech more intelligible. It is intended for students who can already understand and use some English, not for absolute beginners. However, the lessons are flexible enough to be used by high-beginning, intermediate, and low-advanced English as a second or foreign language (ESL/EFL) classes. The material in this book is especially suitable for use in pronunciation, listening and speaking, and oral communication courses, and provides an important balance in integrated skills language courses.

The activities in *Phrase by Phrase* are presented as a systematically organized program to help learners develop auditory sensitivity and improve accuracy, fluency, and confidence in their oral production of English. Listening precedes speaking, for only after hearing and distinguishing sounds can learners be expected to work on improving production. Sounds and sound patterns are presented in the context of connected discourse, rather than as lists of isolated words and sentences, as is frequently done in pronunciation texts. Pronunciation notes are simple but informative, and the teacher is encouraged to add verbal, visual, and kinesthetic explanations to aid the students' mastery of oral production. The activities in each lesson, all of which require active student involvement, are based on a brief narrative, dialog, or expository passage of general interest. The organization of each lesson takes the shape of an hourglass, moving from holistic, or general, to specific listening tasks, and then from specific to holistic pronunciation tasks. Students are guided to listen to and monitor their own progress and make corrections in their pronunciation. They are further encouraged to improve their oral production beyond the repetition of the instructional material.

LISTENING

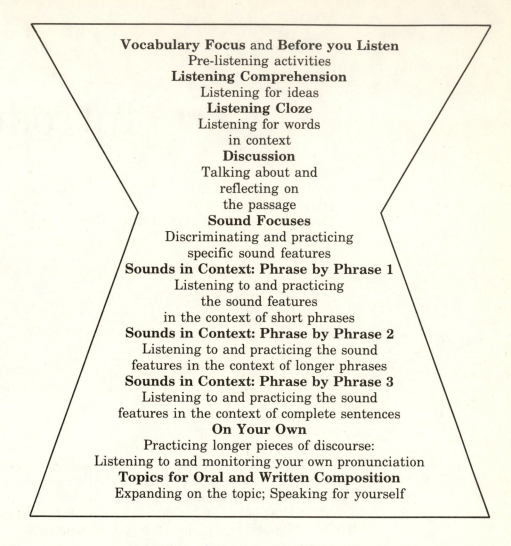

Vocabulary Focus and Before you Listen
Pre-listening activities
Listening Comprehension
Listening for ideas
Listening Cloze
Listening for words
in context
Discussion
Talking about and
reflecting on
the passage
Sound Focuses
Discriminating and practicing
specific sound features
Sounds in Context: Phrase by Phrase 1
Listening to and practicing
the sound features
in the context of short phrases
Sounds in Context: Phrase by Phrase 2
Listening to and practicing the sound
features in the context of longer phrases
Sounds in Context: Phrase by Phrase 3
Listening to and practicing the sound
features in the context of complete sentences
On Your Own
Practicing longer pieces of discourse:
Listening to and monitoring your own pronunciation
Topics for Oral and Written Composition
Expanding on the topic; Speaking for yourself

SPEAKING

Phrase by Phrase introduces stress, intonation, reduction, and linking from
the beginning of the text, and reinforces and expands upon these features at
graduated levels throughout. Understanding and producing the suprasemen-
tal features, which are paramount in giving English its distinct rhythm and
melody and in making pronunciation intelligible, is a necessity for learners
from all language backgrounds. Vowel and consonant groups are presented
alternately throughout the text, and the teacher should focus on those which
are particularly troublesome for learners from certain language backgrounds.
Sound features introduced in one lesson are often used as reference points for
those introduced in subsequent lessons.

The sixteen lessons are graduated in difficulty of vocabulary and syntax
from beginning to end, and shift from concrete topics of a conversational or
narrative mode to abstract topics of an expository nature. Vocabulary is spi-
raled: words and phrases introduced in one lesson may appear in subsequent
lessons. Despite this sequencing, *Phrase by Phrase* allows the teacher the
flexibility to choose the lessons and learning activities which are most appropriate for the students.

The four 90-minute audiotapes for *Phrase by Phrase* form an integral
part of the learning program. The tapes are best used in a pronunciation class

setting with the teacher controlling the pacing, pauses, and repetitions. They are also suitable for use in a teacher-controlled pronunciation laboratory class, and they may be used for individual student practice *after* presentation by the teacher.

For information on videotapes, please contact the author (see the Instructor's Manual for details).

All new words and phrases presented in the Vocabulary Focus sections are listed with their pronunciations in the Pronouncing Glossary at the end of the text. The pronunciations listed are those used in the taped material and those considered most frequently used in the *American Heritage Dictionary*, *Webster's New World Dictionary*, or the *Longman Dictionary of American English*. The phonetic notations in *Phrase by Phrase* use a modified form of the International Phonetic Alphabet, as shown in the Pronunciation Key.

The Instructor's Manual includes a detailed description of the activities, suggestions for their use, and an answer key.

ACKNOWLEDGMENTS

I am grateful to many people for their help in realizing this text-tape project. Sincere thanks and appreciation go to the following: my colleagues across America for reading the manuscript, field-testing portions of it, and offering their constructive criticism[1]; the hundreds of students who used and offered comments on the material as it evolved; Ellen Sasaki, for providing the lively illustrations; my Department Chair, Jo Ford, for her wisdom, humor, and continued encouragement; my Dean of Instruction, Nancy Renkiewicz, for her particular support of the videotape project; the Instructional Design Services staff at Mission College for their assistance and expertise in the audiotaping and videotaping; the students who took part in the audiotaping and videotaping; my editors, Brenda White of Prentice-Hall, and Ann Mohan of Word-Crafters, for their expertise and guidance. I would like to extend special thanks to my family, who offered their unflagging support, encouragement, and understanding throughout this project.

M. J. C.
Santa Clara, California

---

[1]See the Instructor's Manual for a complete list.

Chapter 1

The Grasshopper and the Ants

VOCABULARY FOCUS

Do you or your classmates know the words in this list? Complete each sentence with a word or phrase from the list. Discuss your choices with a partner.

ant	finally	reply	suffer
beautiful	gaze	right	summer
cloudy	grasshopper	starving	
enjoy	pay attention	store	

1. A _____ is an insect which can jump high and make a sharp noise by rubbing parts of its body together.

2. An _____ is a small insect living on the ground and famous for hard work.

3. To be _____ is to be very, very hungry.

4. To _____ is to answer.

5. To _____ is to look steadily.

6. To _____ is to like.

7. A _____ is a privilege.

8. A _____ is a supply.

9. _____ is at last.

10. _____ is the opposite of sunny.

11. _____ is the opposite of ugly.

12. _____ is the opposite of winter.

13. _____ is the opposite of recover.

14. _____ is the opposite of ignore.

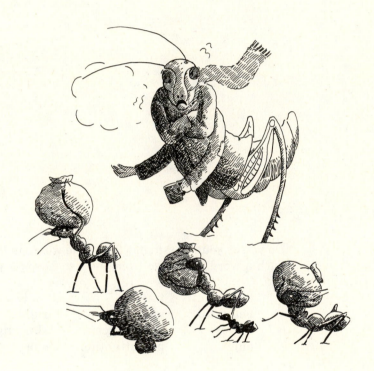

BEFORE YOU LISTEN

Look at the picture and tell what you think.

What are the ants carrying?
Describe the grasshopper's clothing.
What is the grasshopper doing with its arms?

The Grasshopper and the Ants is one of the many fables written by Aesop, a Greek fable writer of the late sixth century B.C. A fable is a story that teaches a lesson, called a *moral*. In a fable animals usually speak and act like human beings. Fables are passed down from generation to generation since their morals are usually timeless. As they relate to human behavior in general, Aesop's fables are known around the world.

LISTENING COMPREHENSION

Read these statements. Listen to the passage and choose the best answer for each statement.

1. The ants were _____ some food.
   - a. drying out
   - b. trying out
   - c. eating
   - d. storing

2. The ants _____ the grasshopper.
   - a. welcomed
   - b. ignored
   - c. laughed at
   - d. gazed at

3. The grasshopper was _____.
   - a. tired
   - b. sick
   - c. angry
   - d. hungry

4. The grasshopper had spent last summer _____.
   - a. eating and dancing
   - b. eating and drinking
   - c. dancing and singing
   - d. dancing and thinking

5. The ants gave the grasshopper _____.
   - a. some money
   - b. a drink
   - c. some food
   - d. nothing

6. a. The ants had worked hard and the grasshopper had, too.
   - b. The ants had worked hard but the grasshopper hadn't.
   - c. The grasshopper had worked hard but the ants hadn't.
   - d. The grasshopper hadn't worked hard and the ants hadn't, either.

LISTENING CLOZE

Listen to the passage again. Fill in the words you hear, one word for each blank. Pause the tape as necessary.

On a (1) _____ sunny winter day

(2) _____ ants had their winter store of food out to

(3) _____. A grasshopper came by and

(4) _____ hungrily at the food. As the ants paid no

(5) _____ to him, he finally said,

"(6) _____ you please give me something to eat?

I'm (7) _____."

"Didn't you (8) _____ away food last summer

(9) _____ use now?" asked the ants.

"No," (10) _____ the grasshopper. "I was

(11) _____ busy enjoying myself and dancing

(12) _____ singing."

"Well, then," said the (13) _____, "live this

winter on (14) _____ dancing and singing, as

(15) _____ live on what we did. No one has a

(16) _____ to play (17) _____

the time, or he'll have to (18) _____ for it."

DISCUSSION

What is the moral of the story?
Why has this story lasted for so many centuries?
Is there a story like this one in your language?

SOUND FOCUS 1: SYLLABLES

A. Every word in English has at least one basic spoken part called a **syllable.** A syllable consists of a single pulse of breath (a beat). A syllable has one vowel sound. It may have one or more consonant sounds, too.[1] Listen to the following words and notice how many syllables each word has. Each dot (·) represents one syllable.

care	careful	carefully
act	react	reaction

B. Listen to the following words. For each syllable, make one of these motions with your hand: (Your teacher may suggest one.)

(a) clap your hands together,
(b) tap one hand on the desk, or
(c) tap one finger on the palm of the other hand

1	2	3	4	5
ant	across	attention	recognizes	refrigerator
food	measure	beautiful	beautifully	pronunciation
taste	absorbed	interact	interaction	vocabulary
bridge	bridges	specific	communicate	communicated

Now read the same list of words aloud. First read down the columns, then read across the rows. While you speak, clap (or tap) once for each syllable.

SOUND FOCUS 2: STRESSED SYLLABLES

A. When a word has two or more syllables, one syllable is **stressed** when spoken. Compared to an unstressed syllable, a *stressed syllable* is *long, strong, clear* and often *high* in tone (or pitch). Listen to these words.

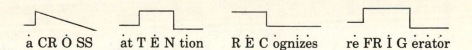

a CR O SS   at T E N tion   R E C ognizes   re FR I G erator

---

[1]A vowel is a sound in which the breath is let out without any stop or any closing of the air passage in the mouth. A consonant is a sound that is made by partly or completely stopping the flow of air as it goes through the mouth.

B. Go back to the list of words in **Sound Focus 1B.** Put a stress mark (ˊ) over the vowel in the most stressed syllable, like this:

    across   attention   recognizes   refrigerator

Rewind the tape and listen to **Sound Focus** 1B again.

SOUND FOCUS 3: UNSTRESSED SYLLABLES
AND REDUCED VOWELS

A. Most two-syllable words have one *stressed* syllable and one **unstressed** syllable. An unstressed syllable has a **reduced vowel.** This vowel is pronounced as the neutral sound /ə/ called a *schwa,* or as a weak /ɪ/. Compared to a stressed syllable, an *unstressed syllable* is *weak, short, unclear* and usually *low* in tone. Listen for the reduced vowels in the following words and draw a line through them.

	Number of clear, stressed vowels	*Number of unclear, reduced vowels*
away	1	1
reply	1	1
common	1	1
remember	1	2
photographer	1	3

B. Although most unstressed syllables have unclear, reduced vowels, some words have unstressed syllables in which the vowel is not reduced. This vowel is clear. However, it is still weaker, shorter, and lower in tone than the clear vowel in a stressed syllable. Listen for the difference between the clear, stressed vowels and the clear, unstressed vowels in each of these words. Underline the clear, stressed syllable.

	Number of clear, stressed vowels	*Number of clear, unstressed vowels*	*Number of unclear, reduced vowels*
decade	1	1	0
concept	1	1	0
backyard	1	1	0

	Number of clear, stressed vowels	Number of clear, unstressed vowels	Number of unclear, reduced vowels
photograph	1	1	1
idea	1	1	1
recognizes	1	1	2
refrigerator	1	1	3

C. Listen for the unclear, reduced vowels in the following words. Draw a line through each reduced vowel.

purpose	phonograph	independent	economical
contain	orchestra	capacity	communicated
sausage	mountainous	geologist	unfortunately

Now read the same list of words aloud. Note that unclear, reduced vowels are never stressed. While you speak, clap (or tap) once for each syllable.

SOUND FOCUS 4: CONTRACTIONS

Words that are spelled with an apostrophe (') in written English may also be reduced in spoken English. The following are some common contractions. The ones in the first column are each one syllable; the vowel in the second, contracted word is deleted. Those in the second column are each two syllables, the vowel in the second, contracted word is reduced to /ə/ or /ɪ/.

1 Syllable	2 Syllables
you're	hasn't
I'm	haven't
it's	hadn't
she's	didn't
we've	it'll
he'd	it'd
I'll	wouldn't
won't	couldn't
don't	shouldn't
can't	mustn't

SOUND FOCUS 5: PHRASE REDUCTIONS

Although they are not contracted in written English, certain verb phrases are greatly reduced in relaxed, informal spoken English.[2] These reductions occur where two words meet, and cause a change in sound. Here are some commonly reduced phrases. Listen first to the full, formal forms, and then to the reduced informal forms. The asterisk (*) before a phrase indicates that it is a *spoken,* but not *written,* reduction.

Going to try	→	*Gonna try
Want to eat.	→	*Wanna eat
Have to suffer	→	*Hafta suffer
Has to try	→	*Hasta try
Got to leave	→	*Gotta leave
Ought to believe	→	*Oughta believe
Did you go?	→	*Didja go?
Would he help?	→	*Woody help?
Won't you play?	→	*Woncha play?
Didn't you know?	→	*Didincha know?

SOUNDS IN CONTEXT: PHRASE BY PHRASE 1

Listen and mark the syllables: put a small dot (·) over each vowel sound in every word. Then rewind the tape and practice the passage in short phrases, marked by the symbol | in the text below.

On a beautiful sunny winter day, | some ants |
had their winter store of food | out to dry. | A grasshopper came by |
and gazed hungrily | at the food. | As the ants |
paid no attention to him, | he finally said, | "Won't you please |
give me something to eat? | I'm starving." |

"Didn't you store away food last summer | for use now?" |
asked the ants. | "No," | replied the grasshopper. | "I was too busy |
enjoying myself | and dancing and singing." |

"Well, then," | said the ants, | "live this winter |
on your dancing and singing, | as we live on what we did. |
No one has a right | to play all the time, | or he'll have to suffer for it."

---

[2]Reductions commonly consist of an auxiliary verb plus an infinitive, or an auxiliary verb plus a pronoun.

SOUNDS IN CONTEXT: PHRASE BY PHRASE 2

Listen and underline the clear vowel sounds. Then rewind the tape and practice the passage in longer phrases, marked by the symbol | in the text below.

On a beautiful sunny winter day, |
some ants had their winter store of food out to dry. |
A grasshopper came by | and gazed hungrily at the food. |
As the ants paid no attention to him, | he finally said, |
"Won't you please give me something to eat? | I'm starving." |
    "Didn't you store away food last summer for use now?" |
asked the ants. | "No," replied the grasshopper. |
"I was too busy enjoying myself | and dancing and singing." |
    "Well, then," said the ants, |
"live this winter on your dancing and singing, |
as we live on what we did. | No one has a right to play all the time, |
or he'll have to suffer for it."

SOUNDS IN CONTEXT: PHRASE BY PHRASE 3

Listen and underline the contractions and phrase reductions. Then rewind the tape and practice the passage in complete sentences, marked by the symbol | in the text below.

On a beautiful sunny winter day, some ants had their winter

store of food out to dry. | A grasshopper came by and gazed hungrily

at the food. | As the ants paid no attention to him, he finally said,

"Won't you please give me something to eat? | I'm starving." |

    "Didn't you store away food last summer for use now?"

asked the ants. | "No," replied the grasshopper. | "I was too busy

enjoying myself and dancing and singing." |

    "Well, then," said the ants, "live this winter

on your dancing and singing, as we live on what we did. |

No one has a right to play all the time, or he'll have to suffer for it."

ON YOUR OWN

Review the **Sound Focus** exercises introduced in this lesson.
Practice the **Phrase by Phrase** steps several times.
Record the passage from beginning to end without stopping.

On a beautiful sunny winter day,

some ants had their winter store of food out to dry.

A grasshopper came by and gazed hungrily at the food.

As the ants paid no attention to him, he finally said,

"Won't you please give me something to eat? I'm starving."

"Didn't you store away food last summer for use now?"

asked the ants." "No," replied the grasshopper.

"I was too busy enjoying myself and dancing and singing."

"Well, then," said the ants,

"live this winter on your dancing and singing,

as we live on what we did. No one has a right to play all the time,

or he'll have to suffer for it."

Listen to your recording.

Did you say the correct number of syllables?
Did you stress the correct syllable in each word?
Did you distinguish between clear and reduced vowels?
Did you reduce the phrases "won't you" to "*woncha,"
"didn't you" to "*didincha," and "have to" to "*hafta"?
In which of these areas do you need to improve?
In what other areas do you need to improve?

TOPICS FOR ORAL OR WRITTEN COMPOSITION

1. Describe an experience of yours, or someone else's, that illustrates the moral of this story.
2. Tell another fable that illustrates a different moral.
3. Point out the characteristics and activities of ants. Explain why ants were used in this fable to represent hard workers.

Chapter 2

Liz's Exercise Program

VOCABULARY FOCUS

Do you or your classmates know the words in this list? Complete each sentence with a word or phrase from the list. Change nouns and verbs to appropriate forms. Discuss your choices with a partner.

cereal	juicy	rotate	stretch
chest	push-up	sausage	sweat
exercise	realize	shoulder	thick
go on a diet	relax	sit-up	toast
jogging			

1. These oranges look too dry. Let's buy those
   _____ ones.

2. Do you like to sit down and _____ after a
   hard day's work?

3. The opposite of *thin* is _____.

4. To make _____, you heat a slice of bread on
   both sides.

5. A _____ is a kind of food made by filling a
   long, eatable tube with very finely chopped meat and spices.

6. Some people eat hot _____, such as oatmeal, for breakfast.

7. Doing _____ every day will help keep you healthy.

8. The upper front part of the body is called the _____.

9. The arms are connected to the _____.

10. To do a _____, you lie on the ground with your face down and then push your body up with your arm muscles.

11. To do a _____, you lie on the ground with your face up, and then you use your stomach muscles to sit up.

12. I like to _____ when I get out of bed. I put my arms up and then straighten my body.

13. _____ is faster than walking and slower than running.

14. In order to lose weight, people often _____.

15. You can _____ a bicycle wheel with your hand. Then the wheel goes around and around.

16. When you are very hot or nervous, _____ comes out from the body through the skin; this water is also called perspiration.

17. I had such a nice time talking with my friend that I didn't _____ how late it was.

BEFORE YOU LISTEN

Look at the picture and tell what you think.

What kind of clothing is Liz wearing?
What kind of exercises is she doing?
What is she having for breakfast?

Americans are concerned about their health and about their figure, or body shape. Especially in the cities, where many jobs do not require physical labor, people try to keep healthy by following an exercise program. Many Americans consider themselves overweight and try to lose weight by going on a diet. Sometimes they succeed, and sometimes they don't!

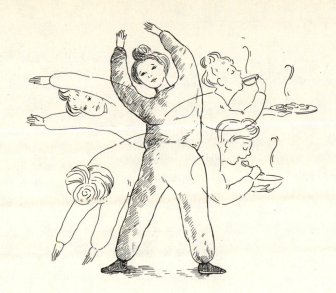

LISTENING COMPREHENSION

Read these statements. Listen to the passage and choose the best answer for each statement.

1. Liz raises her knees to her _____.
   a. chin   c. chest
   b. cheeks   d. neck

2. She stretches her _____.
   a. arms and legs   c. neck and shoulders
   b. hands and feet   d. back and sides

3. She twists her body _____.
   a. from hand to foot   c. from head to toe
   b. from time to time   d. from side to side

4. Liz jogs for _____.
   a. an hour   c. forty minutes
   b. thirteen minutes   d. half an hour

5. As she runs, _____.
   a. she sweats   c. her heart beats fast
   b. she breathes deeply   d. all of the above

6. While jogging, Liz thinks about _____.
   a. seeing her boyfriend c. eating breakfast
   b. losing weight   d. running fast

7. For breakfast she has three _____.
   a. thick sausages   c. fried eggs
   b. cups of coffee   d. juicy oranges

8. Now she must _____.
   a. go for a walk   c. go jogging
   b. go to work   d. go on a diet

LISTENING CLOZE

Listen to the passage again. Fill in the words you hear, one word for each blank. Pause the tape as necessary.

When Liz (1) _____ out of bed at six, she starts doing her (2) _____ right away. First she stretches her arms and (3) _____, and rotates her hands and feet, and (4) _____ her neck and shoulders. She twists her body from side to side, (5) _____ down and touches her toes, and then raises her knees to her (6) _____.

After she does some push-ups and (7) _____, she puts on her shoes and goes jogging. While she (8) _____ for thirty minutes, Liz thinks about (9) _____ weight. As she runs, she (10) _____ deeply, her heart beats fast, and (11) _____ drips from her body. "How healthy this is!" she (12) _____ proudly. When she (13) _____ back home, she takes a shower and (14) _____. Then she goes into the kitchen and fixes breakfast. She (15) _____ two juicy oranges, three fried eggs, four bowls of (16) _____ and five thick (17) _____. She drinks two (18) _____ of coffee and three glasses of milk. Suddenly she (19) _____ what she has done. "Oh, no!" she cries. "Look at my stomach! Now I have to go (20) _____ a diet!"

DISCUSSION

Do you think Miss Jones's exercise program is successful?
What kind of exercises do you do?
What do you have for breakfast?
Would you personally like to lose weight or gain weight?

SOUND FOCUS 1: /s/

To produce the sound /s/, as in *side*, force a hissing, voiceless sound[1] through a narrow opening between your tongue and the upper gum ridge. Underline the letters that make the /s/ sound.

some	Miss	juicy	sweat
side	this	recent	small
sit-up	since	listen	stomach
sausage	six	dancing	spot

SOUND FOCUS 2: /z/

To produce the sound /z/, as in *zoo,* place your teeth and tongue in the same position as for /s/. Force a buzzing, voiced sound through the narrow opening between your tongue and the upper gum ridge. Underline the letters that make the /z/ sound.

zoo	lazy	buzz
zero	losing	is
zip	easy	Ms.
zone	design	realize

SOUND FOCUS 3: SYLLABLES AND WORD STRESS

A. Listen to these words. Mark each syllable by putting a small dot (·) over the vowel sound.

shoulders	oranges	stretches
healthy	stomach	rotates
diet	realizes	exercises

B. Draw the intonation pattern over the above words.

shoulders

---

[1] A *voiceless* sound is made without letting the vocal cords vibrate. A *voiced* sound is made by letting the vocal cords vibrate. Test yourself by placing your fingers on your throat. You will feel your vocal cords vibrating when you say a voiced sound, but not when you say a voiceless sound. To test yourself in another way, cover your ears with your hands. For a voiced sound, you will hear your whole head vibrating.

SOUND FOCUS 4: THIRD PERSON SINGULAR VERB ENDINGS

A. Third person singular present tense verb forms end in the single sounds /s/ or /z/, or an extra syllable /ɪz/, or /əz/.[2] Regular plural noun forms and possessive forms also end in one of these three sounds.

1. /s/		2. /z/		3. /ɪz/	
jump	jumps	jog	jogs	fix	fixes
rotate	rotates	do	does*	raise	raises
put	puts	say	says*	dress	dresses
think	thinks	call	calls	relax	relaxes
sit-up	sit-ups	egg	eggs	glass	glasses
minute	minutes	hand	hands	sausage	sausages
sock	socks	toe	toes	exercise	exercises
Pat	Pat's	Nancy	Nancy's	Max	Max's
Jack	Jack's	Jim	Jim's	Liz	Liz's

*Note the vowel change from base form to third person singular form.

B. Circle the s ending sound (/s/, /z/, or /ɪz/) of each of the following words.

runs	/s, ⓩ, ɪz/	dishes	/s, z, ɪz/
rushes	/s, z, ɪz/	bends	/s, z, ɪz/
takes	/s, z, ɪz/	goes	/s, z, ɪz/
arms	/s, z, ɪz/	touches	/s, z, ɪz/
oranges	/s, z, ɪz/	starts	/s, z, ɪz/
push-ups	/s, z, ɪz/	drips	/s, z, ɪz/

SOUND FOCUS 5: LINKING AND REDUCTION

In writing, words are separated by blank spaces:

She jumps out of bed.

However, in spoken English, words belonging to the same phrase or thought group are **linked,** or joined, together. To learners of English, they are pronounced as if they were all one word:

*Shejumpsoutabed.[3]

---

[2]If the base verb or noun ends in one of the six sibilant or affricate consonants, /s, z, ʃ, ʒ, tʃ, dʒ/, it is pronounced as an extra syllable, /ɪz/ or /əz/. If it ends in any other voiced sound, the ending is pronounced only as the added sound of voiced /z/; if it ends in any other voiceless sound, the ending is pronounced only as the added sound of voiceless /s/.

To help with the concept of linking, try this mental picture. Imagine cubes of ice falling one by one; words spoken one by one are like these ice cubes. Now imagine water flowing smoothly; words linked together in phrases are like this water. Melt the ice cubes into water by letting your breath and voice carry the sound at the end of one word into the sound at the beginning of the next word.

A. Practice shifting the consonant at the end of the first word to the beginning of the next word.

an orange	→ *anorange	think about	→ *thinkabout
all over	→ *allover	look after	→ *lookafter
turn on	→ *turnon	jumps out	→ *jumpsout
leave out	→ *leavout	puts on	→ *putson
take off	→ *takoff	goes into	→ *goezinto
put away	→ *putaway	his own	→ *hizown

B. When the word *and* is used in a phrase, it is usually reduced to /ənd/, /ən/, or simply /n/, or *'n'. The preceding and following sounds are linked to it. The word *of* is usually reduced to /əv/ before a vowel sound and, in relaxed speech, /ə/ before a consonant sound. The word *or* becomes /ɚ/, and the word *at* becomes /ət/ or /ɪt/. Practice linking the words in these phrases.

arms and legs	→ *arms'n'legs
push-ups and sit-ups	→ *pushups'n'sittups
lots of oranges	→ *lotsavoranges
cups of coffee	→ *cupsacoffee
pen or pencil	→ *pennerpencil
up or down	→ *upperdown
look at us	→ *lookitus
look at Ellen	→ *lookitellen

---

[3]The asterisk (*) indicates that the phrase is a *spoken,* but not *written,* form.

SOUNDS IN CONTEXT: PHRASE BY PHRASE 1

Listen and underline the extra syllable /ɪz/. Note that most, but not all, **es** spellings are pronounced as an extra syllable.

Extra syllable: exerci<u>ses</u>   Liz'<u>s</u>

Not an extra syllable: comes

Then rewind the tape and practice the passage in short phrases, marked by the symbol | in the text below.

When Liz | jumps out of bed at six, | she starts doing |
her exercises | right away. | First | she stretches her arms and legs, |
rotates her hands and feet, | and relaxes her neck and shoulders. |
She twists her body | from side to side, |
bends down and touches her toes, | and then raises her knees |
to her chest. | After she does | some push-ups and sit-ups, |
she puts on her shoes | and goes jogging. | While she jogs |
for thirty minutes, | Liz thinks about losing weight. | As she runs, |
she breathes deeply, | her heart beats fast, |
and sweat drips from her body. | "How healthy this is!" |
she says proudly. | When she gets back home, | she takes a shower |
and dresses. | Then she goes into the kitchen | and fixes breakfast. |
She eats two juicy oranges, | three fried eggs, | four bowls of cereal, |
and five thick sausages. | She drinks two cups of coffee |
and three glasses of milk. | Suddenly she realizes | what she has done. |
"Oh, no!" | she cries. | "Look at my stomach! |
Now I have to go on a diet!" |

SOUNDS IN CONTEXT: PHRASE BY PHRASE 2

Listen and underline the /s/ sounds once and the /z/ sounds twice. Note that /s/ sounds can be written with **s**, **c** or **x**, and /z/ sounds can be written with **z** or **s**.

When Li<u><u>z</u></u> jump<u>s</u> out of bed at <u>six</u>,

Then rewind the tape and practice the passage in longer phrases, marked by the symbol | in the text below.

When Liz jumps out of bed at six, |
she starts doing her exercises right away. |
First she stretches her arms and legs, | rotates her hands and feet, |
and relaxes her neck and shoulders. |
She twists her body from side to side, |
bends down and touches her toes, |
and then raises her knees to her chest. |
After she does some push-ups and sit-ups, |
she puts on her shoes and goes jogging. |

While she jogs for thirty minutes, | Liz thinks about losing weight. |
As she runs, she breathes deeply, | her heart beats fast, |
and sweat drips from her body. | "How healthy this is!" |
she says proudly. | When she gets back home, |
she takes a shower and dresses. | Then she goes into the kitchen |
and fixes breakfast. | She eats two juicy oranges, three fried eggs, |
four bowls of cereal, and five thick sausages. |
She drinks two cups of coffee | and three glasses of milk. |
Suddenly she realizes | what she has done. | "Oh, no!" she cries. |
"Look at my stomach! | Now I have to go on a diet!" |

SOUNDS IN CONTEXT: PHRASE BY PHRASE 3

Listen and mark the consonants linked to vowels that follow.

jumps out of bed at six

Then rewind the tape and practice the passage in complete sentences, marked
by the symbol | in the text below.

When Liz jumps out of bed at six, she starts doing her exercises
right away. | First she stretches her arms and legs,
rotates her hands and feet, and relaxes her neck and shoulders. |
She twists her body from side to side, bends down
and touches her toes, and then raises her knees to her chest. |
After she does some push-ups and sit-ups, she puts on her shoes
and goes jogging. | While she jogs for thirty minutes,
Liz thinks about losing weight. | As she runs, she breathes deeply,
her heart beats fast, and sweat drips from her body. |
"How healthy this is!" she says proudly. | When she gets back home,
she takes a shower and dresses. | Then she goes into the kitchen
and fixes breakfast. | She eats two juicy oranges, three fried eggs,
four bowls of cereal, and five thick sausages. |
She drinks two cups of coffee and three glasses of milk. |
Suddenly she realizes what she has done. | "Oh, no!" she cries. |
"Look at my stomach! | Now I have to go on a diet!" |

ON YOUR OWN

Review the **Sound Focus** exercises introduced in this lesson.
Practice the **Phrase by Phrase** steps several times.
Record the passage from beginning to end without stopping.

When Liz jumps out of bed at six, she starts doing her exercises

right away. First she stretches her arms and legs,

rotates her hands and feet, and relaxes her neck and shoulders.

She twists her body from side to side, bends down

and touches her toes, and then raises her knees to her chest.

After she does some push-ups and sit-ups,

she puts on her shoes and goes jogging. While she jogs

for thirty minutes, Liz thinks about losing weight. As she runs,

she breathes deeply, her heart beats fast,

and sweat drips from her body. "How healthy this is!"

she says proudly. When she gets back home, she takes a shower

and dresses. Then she goes into the kitchen and fixes breakfast.

She eats two juicy oranges, three fried eggs, four bowls of cereal,

and five thick sausages. She drinks two cups of coffee

and three glasses of milk. Suddenly she realizes what she has done.

"Oh no!" she cries. "Look at my stomach! Now I have to go on a diet!"

Listen to your recording.

Did you say the correct number of syllables?
Did you pronounce the sounds /s/, /z/, and /ɪz/ clearly?
Did you link words and shift consonants to the next word?
In which of these areas do you need to improve?

TOPICS FOR ORAL OR WRITTEN COMPOSITION

1. Interview a classmate or other friend and find out what process he or she follows to study, cook, clean house, repair a car, buy clothes, or make an important decision. Then describe this process using third person singular verb forms.

2. Describe the duties of a particular job—an office manager, a book-keeper, a computer operator, a coal miner, etc. Give a description of a job that you know about, or look in the classified advertisements of the newspaper for a job that interests you. Use third person singular verb forms.

Chapter 3

What's for Dinner?

VOCABULARY FOCUS

Do you or your classmates know the words in this list? Complete each sentence with a word or phrase from the list. Change nouns and verbs to appropriate forms. Discuss your choices with a partner.

be good at	matter	refrigerator	stuff
chop	mushroom	restaurant	wrap
chopsticks	practically	skin	would rather
dumpling	prawn	soy sauce	yeah
feel like			

1. A _____ is a large box used to keep food cold.

2. To _____ means to cut into small bits with a knife.

3. A _____ is a small piece of steamed or boiled dough served with meat or soup.

4. It doesn't _____ if the pen you use is black or blue, as long as it writes.

5. A _____ is a kind of seafood like shrimp.

6. The thin outer layer of the body or of an object is the _____.

7. _____ is a dark, salty sauce made from soy beans. It's often used in Chinese and other East Asian cooking.

8. I'd prefer to have Italian food, but Lee _____ have Vietnamese food.

9. A _____ is a kind of plant that's good to eat. It is shaped like a little umbrella.

10. Before giving a gift to my friend, I'm going to _____ it in pretty paper.

11. Eating at a _____ is usually more expensive than eating at home.

12. _____ are two small sticks held together in one hand and used in China and other East Asian countries for eating.

13. _____ means the material of which something is made. It is also an informal way to talk about things in a mass or group.

14. Since John _____ playing soccer, he was selected to join the school soccer team.

15. If a container is almost empty, it is _____ empty.

16. I _____ having some ice cream. Do you want some too?

17. An informal way to say *Yes* is _____.

BEFORE YOU LISTEN

Look at the picture and tell what you think.

Where are Mei and Rosa?
What kind of book is Mei holding?
What is going into the big pot on the stove?

Mei and Rosa are roommates. They share an apartment and often plan meals and other activities together. In this dialog they are discussing plans for tonight's dinner.

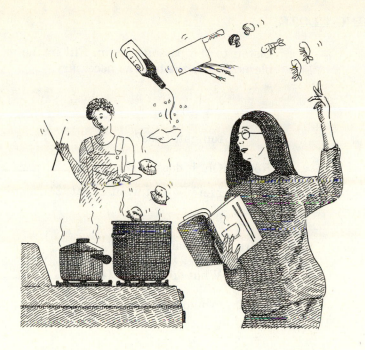

LISTENING COMPREHENSION

Read these statements. Listen to the passage and choose the best answer for each statement.

1. Mei asks Rosa _____ they should eat.
   a. whether   c. where
   b. what   d. when

2. Rosa doesn't _____.
   a. want to eat dinner   c. care what they have for dinner
   b. know how to cook   d. want to think about dinner

3. Rosa and Mei have _____ food at home now.
   a. a lot of   c. hardly any
   b. some   d. no

4. Rosa prefers to have _____ food tonight.
   a. Chinese   c. American
   b. Mexican   d. Japanese

5. Mei makes won ton with _____.
   a. pork, green onions, and black mushrooms
   b. beef, prawns, and green onions
   c. prawns, soy sauce, and carrots
   d. chicken, prawns, and pork

6. Rosa probably thinks it is hardest to _____.
   a. cook   c. wash dishes
   b. chop everything up   d. use chopsticks

LISTENING CLOZE

Listen to the passage again. Fill in the words you hear, one word for each blank. Pause the tape as necessary.

Mei: What (1) _____ you want to have for dinner tonight, Rosa?

Rosa: Oh, it doesn't (2) _____ to me. How about you, Mei? Do you want to eat (3) _____ home or go out?

Mei: Let's eat at home.

Rosa: What do you feel (4) _____ making?

Mei: Would you (5) _____ have Chinese or American food?

Rosa: How about Chinese food?

Mei: Okay, we can make *won ton*—you know, meat (6) _____ in soup?

Rosa: Yeah, that sounds great.

Mei: The refrigerator is (7) _____ empty. We'll have to buy some pork, (8) _____, green onions, and black mushrooms. And we'll need some won ton (9) _____, soy sauce, and chicken bones.

Rosa: Will we have to (10) _____ everything up into little pieces?

Mei: Just the (11) _____ that has to go into the filling.

Rosa: Will it take long to (12) _____ the dumplings?

Mei: Well, how good are you (13) _____ using chopsticks?

Rosa: Chopsticks? You mean I (14) _____ to use chopsticks?

Mei: Why, of (15) _____!

Rosa: I have a better (16) _____. Let's go to a restaurant for dinner.

Mei: Why?

Rosa: Well, uh, we (17) _____ have to wash dishes.

DISCUSSION

Do people eat dumplings where you come from?

What kind of food do you usually eat? Do you like to cook?

Do you have a roommate? What do you and your roommate do together?

SOUND FOCUS 1: RISING AND FALLING INTONATION

A. **Intonation** refers to the rise and fall in the level, or pitch, of the voice. Hearing intonation is important in determining meaning. Likewise, using proper intonation is important in expressing your meaning correctly. In the following examples, the word or phrase is said first with *even* intonation. Then, it is repeated with *rising* intonation, which asks a question, and finally, with *falling* intonation, which makes a statement or response.

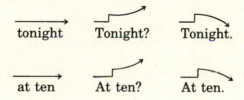

B. Listen to these letters of the alphabet and mark the intonation you hear: rising or falling.

A?   B?   C?   D.   E.   F.

G?   H.   I?   J?   K.   L.

Now practice saying the letters, one at a time, to a partner. Have your partner tell you whether he or she hears rising or falling intonation.

SOUND FOCUS 2: STATEMENT INTONATION

A. Spoken sentences usually follow certain intonation patterns.[1] For statements (both affirmative and negative), the voice starts at a middle level tone, rises to a higher level on the stressed syllable of the last stressed word, and falls to a low tone at the end. Listen to the rise-falling pattern.

---

[1]Note that not all speakers use the same intonation, and even the same speaker does not always use the exact same intonation. However, the patterns presented are generally used by speakers of American English.

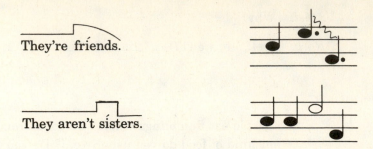

They're friends.

They aren't sisters.

Note that in the one-syllable word *friends,* the voice glides down. Since the word *sister* has more than one syllable, the voice steps down.

B. First listen and mark the intonation pattern of the sentences below. Then practice saying them to a partner.

Let's eat at home.

That sounds great.

I have a better idea.

SOUND FOCUS 3: YES/NO QUESTION INTONATION

A. In questions that have a *yes* or *no* answer, the voice commonly rises to a higher level at the end.

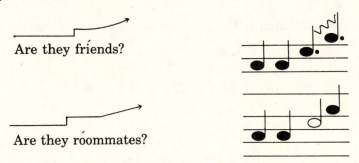

Are they friends?

Are they roommates?

Note again that in the one-syllable word *friends,* the voice glides up, while in the word *roommates,* which has two syllables, the voice steps up.

B. First listen and mark the intonation pattern of the *Yes/No* questions below. Then practice saying them to a partner.

Are you hungry?

Do you know how to cook?

Won't you give me some food?

SOUND FOCUS 4: WH– QUESTION INTONATION

A. Information questions beginning with *Who, What, Where, When, Why, Which, How,* etc. follow the same rising-falling intonation pattern as statements. Listen to the intonation in these **WH- questions.**

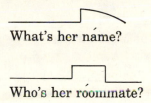

What's her name?

Who's her roommate?

B. First listen and mark the intonation pattern of the questions below. Then practice saying them to a partner.

How about you?

What do you want to make?

How good are you at using chopsticks?

SOUND FOCUS 5: CHOICE QUESTION INTONATION

A. Some questions give the responder a choice. **Choice** questions use the word *or* between two parts of the question. The first part of the question uses the rising intonation of a *Yes/No* question, and the second part of the question uses the falling intonation of a statement.

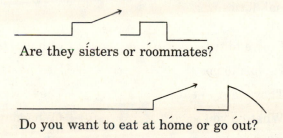

Are they sisters or roommates?

Do you want to eat at home or go out?

B. First listen and mark the intonation pattern of the questions below. Then practice saying them to a partner.

Would you rather have Chinese or American food?

Is the refrigerator empty or full?

Do you want to use chopsticks or a fork?

SOUND FOCUS 6: LISTING INTONATION

A. When listing several items, the first few are usually spoken with a rising intonation. The last item, which comes after the words *and* or *or,* is spoken with falling intonation. Listen to the **listing intonation** in these phrases.

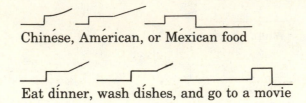

Chinese, American, or Mexican food

Eat dinner, wash dishes, and go to a movie

B. First listen and mark the intonation pattern of the phrases below. Then practice saying them to a partner.

A fork, a knife, and a spoon

Listening, thinking, and speaking

A red one, a yellow one, and a green one

SOUND FOCUS 7: REDUCTIONS: *HAFTA, *HASTA,
**   *WANNA, *WHADDAYA,**
**   *KIN**

The phrases *have to* and *has to,* meaning *must,* are commonly reduced to *hafta* and *hasta* in relaxed, informal speech. The phrase *want to* is often reduced to *wanna,* the phrases *What are you* or *What do you* to *Whaddaya,* and the word *can* to *kin.* The two roommates in this dialog, who are speaking in a relaxed and informal manner, use these reduced forms.

First practice the full, formal forms. Then practice the reductions in the informal forms.[2]

I have to try.	→ I *hafta try.
He has to go.	→ He *hasta go.
They want to eat.	→ They *wanna eat.
What do you want?	→ *Whaddaya want?
What do you want to have?	→ *Whaddaya *wanna have?
What do you have to do?	→ *Whaddaya *hafta do?
We can see.	→ We *kin see.
She can ask.	→ She *kin ask.
I can do it.	→ I *kin do it.

---

[2]The asterisk (*) indicates that the phrase is a *spoken,* but not *written,* reduction.

SOUNDS IN CONTEXT: PHRASE BY PHRASE 1

Listen and mark the intonation at the end of each phrase. Use short arrows: ↗ for rising, and ↘ for falling, and → for even intonation. Then rewind the tape and practice the passage in short phrases, marked by the symbol | in the text below.

Mei: What do you want to have | for dinner tonight, | Rosa? |

Rosa: Oh, | it doesn't matter | to me. | How about you, | Mei? |

Do you want to eat at home | or go out? |

Mei: Let's eat at home. |

Rosa: What do you feel like making? |

Mei: Would you rather have Chinese | or American food? |

Rosa: How about Chinese food? |

Mei: Okay, | we can make *won ton* | —you know, |

meat dumplings in soup? |

Rosa: Yeah, | that sounds great. |

Mei: The refrigerator | is practically empty. | We'll have to buy |

some pork, | prawns, | green onions | and black mushrooms. |

And we'll need | some won ton skins, | soy sauce, |

and chicken bones. |

Rosa: Will we have to chop everything up | into little pieces? |

Mei: Just the stuff | that has to go | into the filling. |

Rosa: Will it take long | to wrap the dumplings? |

Mei: Well, | how good are you | at using chopsticks? |

Rosa: Chopsticks? | You mean | I have to use chopsticks? |

Mei: Why, | of course! |

Rosa: I have a better idea. | Let's go to a restaurant | for dinner. |

Mei: Why? |

Rosa: Well, | uh, | we won't have to wash dishes. |

SOUNDS IN CONTEXT: PHRASE BY PHRASE 2

Listen and underline the contractions and phrase reductions. Then rewind the tape and practice the passage in complete sentences, marked by the symbol | in the text below.

Mei: What do you want to have for dinner tonight, Rosa? |

Rosa: Oh, it doesn't matter to me. | How about you, Mei? |
          Do you want to eat at home or go out? |

Mei: Let's eat at home. |

Rosa: What do you feel like making? |

Mei: Would you rather have Chinese or American food? |

Rosa: How about Chinese food? |

Mei: Okay, we can make *won ton*—you know, meat dumplings in soup? |

Rosa: Yeah, that sounds great. |

Mei: The refrigerator is practically empty. | We'll have to buy some pork, prawns, green onions and black mushrooms. | And we'll need some won ton skins, soy sauce, and chicken bones. |

Rosa: Will we have to chop everything up into little pieces? |

Mei: Just the stuff that has to go into the filling. |

Rosa: Will it take long to wrap the dumplings? |

Mei: Well, how good are you at using chopsticks? |

Rosa: Chopsticks? | You mean I have to use chopsticks? |

Mei: Why, of course! |

Rosa: I have a better idea. | Let's go to a restaurant for dinner. |

Mei: Why? |

Rosa: Well, uh, we won't have to wash dishes. |

ON YOUR OWN

Review the **Sound Focus** exercises introduced in this lesson.
Practice the **Phrase by Phrase** steps several times.
Record the passage from beginning to end without stopping.

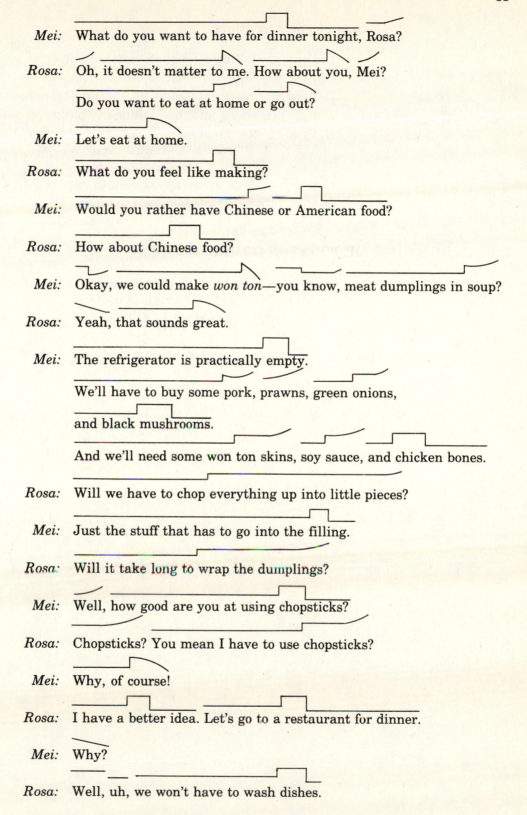

Mei: What do you want to have for dinner tonight, Rosa?

Rosa: Oh, it doesn't matter to me. How about you, Mei?

       Do you want to eat at home or go out?

Mei: Let's eat at home.

Rosa: What do you feel like making?

Mei: Would you rather have Chinese or American food?

Rosa: How about Chinese food?

Mei: Okay, we could make *won ton*—you know, meat dumplings in soup?

Rosa: Yeah, that sounds great.

Mei: The refrigerator is practically empty.

       We'll have to buy some pork, prawns, green onions,

       and black mushrooms.

       And we'll need some won ton skins, soy sauce, and chicken bones.

Rosa: Will we have to chop everything up into little pieces?

Mei: Just the stuff that has to go into the filling.

Rosa: Will it take long to wrap the dumplings?

Mei: Well, how good are you at using chopsticks?

Rosa: Chopsticks? You mean I have to use chopsticks?

Mei: Why, of course!

Rosa: I have a better idea. Let's go to a restaurant for dinner.

Mei: Why?

Rosa: Well, uh, we won't have to wash dishes.

Listen to your recording.

Did you use falling intonation on statements?

Did you use falling intonation on *WH-* questions?

Did you use rising intonation on *Yes/No* questions?

Did you use rising and then falling intonation on choice questions?

Did you reduce the phrases "have to" to "*hafta," "has to" to "*hasta," "want to" to "*wanna," "What do you" to "*Whaddaya," and "can" to "*kin"?

In which of these areas do you need to improve?

In what other areas do you need to improve?

TOPICS FOR ORAL OR WRITTEN COMPOSITION

1. What is your favorite dish? Explain what it tastes, looks and smells like. If possible, tell how it is made.

2. Do you like American food? If so, what kind? Is there any kind you dislike?

3. What are the advantages (or disadvantages) of having a roommate?

Chapter 4

John Thornton's Love for Buck

VOCABULARY FOCUS

Do you or your classmates know the words in this list? Complete each sentence with a word or phrase from the list. Change nouns and verbs to appropriate forms. Discuss your choices with a partner.

can't help	further	name-calling	sparkle
delight	heart	perfect	spring
duty	look after	remain	throat
embrace	master	rough	vibrate

1. Your homework is completely correct. It is

   _____.

2. Another way to say *stay* is _____.

3. The opposite of *smooth* is _____.

4. Ruth was eager for her husband to return. When she heard his

   footsteps, she _____ to her feet to open the door.

5. As soon as she saw her husband, she reached out her arms and gave

   him a big _____.

6. The _____, which is located inside the chest,

   controls the flow of blood through the body. It is also considered to

   be the center of a person's feelings.

7. Will you _____ the baby while I go shopping?

8. When you pronounce the sound /z/, your vocal cords _____, and when you pronounce the sound /s/, they don't.

9. I know I really shouldn't have any more chocolate cake, but it is so delicious that I _____ having just one more slice.

10. The children enjoy playing in the park very much. They respond with great _____ whenever their parents suggest going there.

11. The _____ of these dogs has trained them to behave very well.

12. Johnny's mother told him that it was unkind to say bad or rude things about Billy, and that his _____ would hurt his little friend's feelings.

13. Collecting the monthly rent is one of the _____ of an apartment manager.

14. Look! Diana's diamond ring _____ in the sunlight.

15. Michael has trouble talking today because he has a sore _____.

16. We've talked about this matter a little, and we'll discuss it _____ when we meet again next week.

BEFORE YOU LISTEN

Look at the picture and tell what you think.

Is the man fighting or playing with his dog?
What is the relationship between the man and the dog?
Are the two dogs in the picture the same or different ones?

The Call of the Wild is a novel written by the American author and adventurer, Jack London (1876–1916). The story takes place in the wild north. In this unsettled wilderness, goods are moved through the snow on sleds pulled by dogs. This passage describes the love of John Thornton, the main character, for Buck, one of his sled dogs.[1]

_____
[1]From *The Call of the Wild* by Jack London (New York: Macmillan 1903).

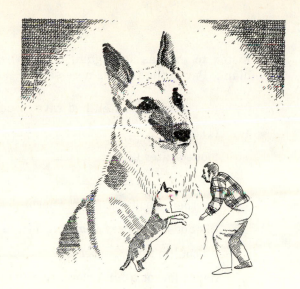

LISTENING COMPREHENSION

Read these statements. Listen to the passage and choose the best answer for each statement.

1. John Thornton looked after his dogs _____.
   a. because they were his duty
   b. because they were his children
   c. as if they were his children
   d. because they had saved his life

2. Other men treated their dogs _____ John Thornton did.
   a. less kindly than   c. more kindly than
   b. as kindly as   d. much more kindly than

3. John Thornton enjoyed talking _____.
   a. about the other men   c. about his dogs
   b. with the other men   d. with his dogs

4. _____ rested his head upon _____.
   a. Buck . . . John Thornton's   c. John Thornton . . . the other men's
   b. Buck . . . the other dogs'   d. John Thornton . . . Buck's

5. John Thornton shook Buck's head _____.
   a. roughly   c. kindly
   b. gently   d. suddenly

6. It seemed Buck's heart would be shaken out of his body because he was _____.
   a. very joyful   c. very angry
   b. very frightened   d. very hurt

7. When John Thornton let go of Buck, Buck _____.
   a. barked loudly   c. jumped up
   b. wagged his tail   d. none of the above

LISTENING CLOZE

Listen to the passage again. Fill in the words you hear, one word for each blank. Pause the tape as necessary.

John Thornton had saved Buck's life; but,

(1) _____, he was the perfect master. Other men

looked after (2) _____ dogs because they

(3) _____ it was their duty and because it was good

for their business. John Thornton (4) _____ after

his dogs as if they were his own (5) _____ because

he couldn't (6) _____ it. And he saw further. He

never forgot a kind word, and to sit down for a long talk

(7) _____ them was his delight as much

(8) _____ theirs. He had a way of taking Buck's

(9) _____ roughly between his hands, and resting

his (10) _____ head upon Buck's. He would shake

Buck back and (11) _____, all the time calling him

bad names, which to Buck were love names. Buck

(12) _____ no greater joy than his master's

(13) _____ embrace and name-calling. At each

(14) _____ back and forth it seemed that his

(15) _____ would be shaken out of his body, for his

joy was so great. And when John Thornton let him go, Buck sprang to

his feet. His (16) _____ laughed, his

(17) _____ sparkled, and his

(18) _____ vibrated with unspoken sounds. In that

manner, Buck remained (19) _____ moving, so that

John Thornton would cry, "God! You (20) _____

almost speak!"

DISCUSSION

If Buck could speak, what do you think he might say?
Have you ever felt the way John Thornton did about an animal?
How do Americans generally treat dogs?

SOUND FOCUS 1: STRESSING CONTENT WORDS

In phrases and sentences, some words are stressed and others are not. Which words in a phrase should be stressed? This depends on what the speaker considers important. However, in general, *content words are stressed* and *function words are unstressed.*

Content words include main verbs, nouns, adjectives, and adverbs. They also include demonstrative pronouns, possessive pronouns, reflexive pronouns, negatives, question words, numbers and quantity words.

Function words include articles, prepositions, conjunctions, auxiliary verbs and personal pronouns. They also include possessive adjectives, relative pronouns, and forms of the verb *be.*

First listen to how the content words, which are underlined, are stronger, longer, clearer, and higher than the other words. Then practice saying these phrases to a partner.

On a beautiful sunny winter day
gazed hungrily at the food
What do you want to have?
Would you rather have Chinese or American food?
She drinks two cups of coffee.
That's not mine.
John Thornton had saved Buck's life.
You can almost speak!

Function words can also be stressed for emphasis, especially for contrast.[2]

It was his delight as much as theirs.

SOUND FOCUS 2: /θ/

A. To produce the sound /θ/, as in *thin,* hold the tip of your tongue loosely between the upper and lower teeth. Let your voiceless breath flow out continuously and smoothly between the top of your tongue and your upper teeth. Keep your lips relaxed.[3]

Underline the letters that make the /θ/ sound.

thin	thought	author	mouth
thick	thumb	nothing	forth
think	Thornton	anything	both
thank	throat	everything	teeth

---

[2]See Lesson 13 for more on contrastive stress and intonation.
[3]When learning to make these and other sounds, it is advisable to use a mirror to reflect the position of your jaw, lips, teeth, and tongue. To check yourself for the /θ/ sound, place your hand in front of your mouth. You can feel a continuous flow of air when you say this sound correctly. To check yourself in another way, hold a small piece of paper in front of your mouth. The paper will bend away from your mouth as long as your breath flows out smoothly.

B. Practice saying these sentences to a partner.

My teeth are in my mouth.
Thank you for everything.
Both Faith and Seth are authors.
Throw the things back and forth.

SOUND FOCUS 3: /ð/.

A. To produce the sound /ð/, as in *this*, hold the tip of your tongue between the teeth, as for /θ/, and make a continuous voiced sound. Do not blow out air.

Underline the letters that make the /ð/ sound.

this	the	other	with*
that	then	further	bathe
these	them	rather	smooth
those	theirs	without*	breathe

With and *without* can be pronounced either /θ/ or /ð/.

B. Practice saying these sentences to a partner.

I'd rather go without them.
There are other ways to bathe.
Breathe deeply and smoothly.
This is their mother and that's their father.

SOUND FOCUS 4: /h/

To produce the sound /h/, as in *house*, relax and open your throat and breathe out air without vibrating your vocal cords. Continue letting out this breath of air as you glide your lips and tongue into position for the following sound.[4]

Underline the letters that make the /h/ sound.

house	heart	ahead
horn	hand	perhaps
head	help	behind

SOUND FOCUS 5: LINKING AND DISAPPEARANCE OF /h/

In informal or rapid speech, unstressed words are reduced. Vowel sounds are shortened and reduced to /ə/ as in the first syllable of the words *ahead* and

---

[4]To check yourself, place your hand in front of your mouth and feel the continuous flow of air. Or, hold a small piece of paper in front of your mouth and watch it move.

behind. Consonant sounds are also changed, as in *woncha and *didincha. When a pronoun or auxiliary verb beginning with the letter **h** is unstressed in spoken English and does not come at the beginning of a phrase, the sound /h/ can disappear completely. Listen for the presence (<u>h</u>) or absence (h̶) of h.

Give h̶er a <u>h</u>ot dog.	*Giver a hotdog.
John h̶ad saved h̶im.	*Johnid savedim.
Will h̶e <u>h</u>ave a <u>h</u>amburger?	⁺Willy hava hamburger?
<u>H</u>elen h̶as <u>h</u>urt h̶erself.	*Heleniz hurterself.
Is h̶e at <u>h</u>ome?	*Izzy at home?

Notice that **h** disappears from unstressed pronouns and auxiliary verbs and is often linked to the last sound in the previous word.

SOUNDS IN CONTEXT: PHRASE BY PHRASE 1

Listen and underline the content words. Also underline two function words that are stressed for contrast. Then rewind the tape and practice the passage in short phrases.

John <u>Thornton</u> had <u>saved</u> <u>Buck's</u> <u>life</u>:| but, <u>further</u>, |
he was the perfect master. | Other men looked after their dogs |
because they thought | it was their duty | and because it was good |
for their business. | John Thornton looked after his dogs |
as if they were his own children, | because he couldn't help it. |
And he saw further. | He never forgot a kind word, | and to sit down |
for a long talk with them | was his delight | as much as theirs. |
He had a way | of taking Buck's head roughly | between his hands, |
and resting his own head | upon Buck's. | He would shake Buck |
back and forth, | all the time calling him bad names, | which to Buck |
were love names. | Buck knew no greater joy |
than his master's rough embrace | and name-calling. |
At each pull back and forth, | it seemed that his heart |
would be shaken out of his body, | for his joy was so great. |
And when John Thornton let him go, | Buck sprang to his feet. |
His mouth laughed, | his eyes sparkled, | and his throat vibrated |
with unspoken sounds. | In that manner |
Buck remained without moving, | so that John Thornton would cry, |
"God! | You can almost speak!" |

SOUNDS IN CONTEXT: PHRASE BY PHRASE 2

Listen and underline the /ð/ sounds once and the /θ/ sounds twice. Then rewind the tape and practice the passage in longer phrases.

John <u>Thornton</u> had saved Buck's life; |
but, fur<u>th</u>er, he was <u>the</u> perfect master. |

Other men looked after their dogs
because they thought it was their duty |
and because it was good for their business. |
John Thornton looked after his dogs as if they were his own children, |
because he couldn't help it. | And he saw further. |
He never forgot a kind word, |
and to sit down for a long talk with them |
was his delight as much as theirs. |
He had a way of taking Buck's head roughly between his hands, |
and resting his own head upon Buck's. |
He would shake Buck back and forth, |
all the time calling him bad names, which to Buck were love names. |
Buck knew no greater joy |
than his master's rough embrace and name-calling. |
At each pull back and forth, |
it seemed that his heart would be shaken out of his body, |
for his joy was so great. | And when John Thornton let him go, |
Buck sprang to his feet. | His mouth laughed, his eyes sparkled, |
and his throat vibrated with unspoken sounds. |
In that manner Buck remained without moving, |
so that John Thornton would cry, | "God! You can almost speak!" |

SOUNDS IN CONTEXT: PHRASE BY PHRASE 3

Listen and underline the /h/ sounds which are pronounced clearly. Draw a
slash (/) through reduced /h/ sounds that have "disappeared." Note that some
h letters are always silent. Cross out (X) an **h** that never makes a sound. Then
rewind the tape and practice the passage in complete sentences.

JoXn Thornton Xad saved Buck's life; but, further,
he was the perfect master. | Other men looked after their dogs
because they thought it was their duty and because it was good for
their business. | John Thornton looked after his dogs
as if they were his own children, because he couldn't help it. |
And he saw further. | He never forgot a kind word, and to sit down
for a long talk with them was his delight as much as theirs. |
He had a way of taking Buck's head roughly between his hands,
and resting his own head upon Buck's. | He would shake Buck
back and forth, all the time calling him bad names, which to Buck
were love names. | Buck knew no greater joy
than his master's rough embrace and name-calling. |
At each pull back and forth, it seemed that his heart
would be shaken out of his body, for his joy was so great. |
And when John Thornton let him go, Buck sprang to his feet. |
His mouth laughed, his eyes sparkled, and his throat vibrated with

unspoken sounds. | In that manner
Buck remained without moving, so that John Thornton would cry,
"God! You can almost speak!" |

ON YOUR OWN

Review the **Sound Focus** exercises introduced in this lesson.
Practice the **Phrase by Phrase** steps several times.
Record the passage from beginning to end without stopping.

John Thornton had saved Buck's life; but, further,
he was the perfect master. Other men looked after their dogs
because they thought it was their duty and because it was good
for their business. John Thornton looked after his dogs
as if they were his own children, because he couldn't help it.
And he saw further. He never forgot a kind word, and to sit down
for a long talk with them was his delight as much as theirs.
He had a way of taking Buck's head roughly between his hands,
and resting his own head upon Buck's. He would shake Buck
back and forth, all the time calling him bad names,
which to Buck were love names. Buck knew no greater joy
than his master's rough embrace and name-calling.
At each pull back and forth, it seemed that his heart
would be shaken out of his body, for his joy was so great.
And when John Thornton let him go, Buck sprang to his feet.
His mouth laughed, his eyes sparkled, and his throat vibrated
with unspoken sounds. In that manner
Buck remained without moving,
so that John Thornton would cry, "God! you can almost speak!"

Listen to your recording.

Did you make the content words long, clear and high?
Did you also lengthen the two stressed pronouns?
Did you pronounce the sounds /θ/ and /ð/ clearly?
Did you make a distinction between /h/ and /h̸/?
In which of these areas do you need to improve?
In what other areas do you need to improve?

TOPICS FOR ORAL OR WRITTEN COMPOSITION

1. Read a story or novel by Jack London. Give a brief summary and tell your impressions of the story.

2. Choose another animal that human beings use to help them work, such as the horse, the ox, or the elephant. Describe the kind of work this kind of animal does.

3. Describe any differences you have noticed between the way dogs are treated by Americans and by people from other countries.

Chapter 5

Cleaning Up
the Backyard

VOCABULARY FOCUS

Do you or your classmates know the words in this list? Complete each sentence with a word or phrase from the list. Change nouns and verbs to appropriate forms. Discuss your choices with a partner.

daisy	inspire	neighbor	shed
fertilizer	kid	patch	tulip
hose	meanwhile	rake	vegetable
impressed	mow	result	weed

1. Carrots, corn, tomatoes, lettuce, and beans are different kinds of

   _____.

2. I use a watering can to water the plants indoors, but a

   _____ to water the lawn outside.

3. If we add some _____ to these plants, they'll probably grow better.

4. The grass in the backyard has grown pretty high. Next weekend I'd better _____ the lawn.

5. I'll also _____ the garden because I don't want those wild plants growing in with the flowers.

6. After the wind stops blowing. I'll go out and
_____ up the leaves.

7. A _____ is a colorful cup-shaped flower;
Holland is famous for growing this kind of flower.

8. A _____ is a flower that has a yellow center
and many white rays around it.

9. How do you make your garden grow so beautifully? I'm
_____ by your green thumb.

10. Your success is a _____ of your skill and your
hard work.

11. I'm not much of a carpenter, but seeing the nice desk and chairs
you've built yourself has _____ me to try to
make some simple bookshelves.

12. Since the roof has a hole in it, rain will leak into it unless we
_____ it.

13. Don't take those dirty garden tools into the house. Keep them in
the _____ behind the house.

14. _____ are people who live nearby.

15. An informal way to refer to a child or a young person is to call
him or her a _____.

16. I waited about ten minutes for the doctor to see me.
_____, I read a magazine.

BEFORE YOU LISTEN

Look at the picture and tell what you think.

Where is the Taylor family? What are they doing?
Is it a weekday or a weekend day?
What kind of plants are growing in the backyard?
What's in the building?

One day the speaker looked out her window and noticed her neighbors cleaning up their backyard. She saw the entire family get involved and how their efforts produced beautiful results.

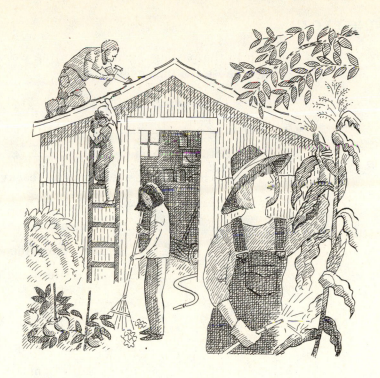

LISTENING COMPREHENSION

Read these statements. Listen to the passage and choose the best answer for each statement.

1. Tina added fertilizer to the _____.
   a. leaves
   b. vegetables
   c. weeds
   d. flowers

2. David is the _____.
   a. mother
   b. father
   c. daughter
   d. son

3. David patched _____.
   a. the whole shed
   b. the hose in the shed
   c. a hole in the roof
   d. a wall in the shed

4. Debbie did not _____.
   a. mow the lawn
   b. plant some tulips
   c. rake up the dead leaves
   d. climb up and down the ladder

5. "Tommy lent a hand" means _____.
   a. Tommy helped
   b. Tommy needed help
   c. Tommy reached with his hand
   d. Tommy took something in his hand

6. The _____ of their day's work was inspiring.
   a. result
   b. resort
   c. reason
   d. resolve

LISTENING CLOZE

Listen to the passage again. Fill in the words you hear, one word for each blank. Pause the tape as necessary.

Tina and David Taylor, my nextdoor

(1) _____, take good care of their home.

On Saturday, I couldn't help (2) _____

their whole family working in the backyard. I guess they

(3) _____ to do a lot of things, because they

(4) _____ pretty early in the morning. Tina

(5) _____ the garden and added fertilizer to the

(6) _____. Her daughter, Debbie,

(7) _____ up the dead leaves and

(8) _____ the lawn. Meanwhile, David

(9) _____ a hole in the roof of the shed. Even

(10) _____ Tommy lent a hand. He

(11) _____ up and down the ladder and got the

tools his father (12) _____. Later, David made a

couple of flower boxes. The kids planted some

(13) _____ and daisies in them. Their mother

(14) _____ some corn and tomatoes and took them

into the house. Then she (15) _____ out the garden

hose and (16) _____ the whole yard. When I

(17) _____ out the window again in the afternoon,

they'd (18) _____ everything. I was so

(19) _____ by the results of their work that it's

(20) _____ me to clean up my own backyard!

DISCUSSION

Do you have a backyard? What do you grow in it?

How do you take care of it?

Have you been so impressed by someone else's work that it has inspired you to do something?

SOUND FOCUS 1: WORD STRESS AND INTONATION

Listen to these words and draw the intonation pattern.

David   results   backyard   started

because   neighbors   fertilizer   impressed

afternoon   vegetables   tomatoes   flower boxes

SOUND FOCUS 2: /t/

A. To produce the stop sound /t/, as in *time,* place the tip of your tongue firmly against the upper gum ridge (above and behind the upper front teeth). This stops the air from flowing out of your mouth. Then blow the tongue away sharply without voice. Be careful not to let the tongue touch the teeth. When pronouncing the sound /t/ at the beginning of a stressed syllable, release a sharp puff of air as you pull your tongue away from the gum ridge.[1]

Underline the letters that make the /t/ sound.

two	turn	return
time	tools	maintain
take	Tommy	attention
tulip	Tina	photography

B. When the sound /t/ comes at the beginning of an unstressed syllable, after the sound /s/, or at the end of a word, do not release a puff of air.

but	today	result
hat	tomato	want
built	fertilizer	start
lent	afternoon	first

C. In American English, when the sound /t/ comes before a reduced vowel and after a stressed or unstressed vowel, it is pronounced as a short voiced sound. To produce this sound, let the tip of your tongue tap the upper gum ridge very quickly.

city	letter	Saturday
writer	forty	automatic
fatter	sit-up	photograph
		(compare with photography)

_____

[1]Test yourself by placing your hand in front of your mouth. You can feel a sudden puff of air when you say this sound correctly. To test yourself in another way, hold a small piece of paper in front of your mouth. The paper will move suddenly when you say this sound correctly.

SOUND FOCUS 3: /d/

To produce the sound /d/, as in <u>d</u>o, place the tip of your tongue against the upper gum ridge, as for the sound /t/. Again, be careful not to let the tongue touch the teeth. Then release the tongue, making a voiced sound. When the sound /d/ comes at the end of a word, do not release the tongue.

Underline the letters that make the /d/ sound.

<u>d</u>o	ladder	made
Debbie	needed	shed
David	window	hard
daisies	garden	kid

Note that the tongue position is the same for the sounds /t/ and /d/. However, for voiceless /t/ at the beginning of a stressed syllable, use your energy in releasing a sharp puff of air, and for voiced /d/, use your energy in vibrating your vocal cords.

SOUND FOCUS 4: REGULAR PAST TENSE ENDINGS

A. Regular past tense and past participle verb forms, written **ed,** end in the single sounds /t/ or /d/, or an extra syllable /əd/ or /ɪd/.[2] Practice the three endings in the following words.

1. /t/		*2. /d/*		*3. /ɪd/*	
rake	raked	mow	mowed	want	wanted
dump	dumped	pull	pulled	hate	hated
patch	patched	turn	turned	start	started
help	helped	climb	climbed	add	added
finish	finished	water	watered	need	needed
impress	impressed	marry	married	weed	weeded

B. Circle the **ed** sound (/t/, /d/, or /ɪd/) of each of the following verbs:

looked	/(t) d, ɪd /	lived	/ t, d, ɪd /
caused	/ t, d, ɪd /	rested	/ t, d, ɪd /
folded	/ t, d, ɪd /	played	/ t, d, ɪd /

---

[2]If the base verb ends in the sound /t/ or /d/, the **ed** ending is pronounced as an extra syllable /əd/ or /ɪd/. If it ends in any voiceless consonant sound except /t/, the ending is pronounced only as the add sound of voiceless /t/. If it ends in a vowel sound or any voiced consonant sound except /d/, the ending is pronounced only as the add sound of voiced /d/.

passed	/ t, d, ɪd /	rafted	/ t, d, ɪd /
carried	/ t, d, ɪd /	flashed	/ t, d, ɪd /
floated	/ t, d, ɪd /	jumped	/ t, d, ɪd /

SOUND FOCUS 5: VOWEL LENGTH

A. The first word in each pair below ends in a voiceless consonant /t/, /s/, or /θ/. The second word ends in a voiced consonant /d/, /z/, or /ð/. Hold the vowel longer when it is followed by a voiced sound.

/-t/	/—d/	/-s/	/—z/	/-θ/	/—ð/
seat	s ee d	ice	eye s	teeth	t ee the
sight	s i de	place	pl ay s	breath	br ea the*
mate	m a de	lace	l ay s	bath	b a the*
kit	k i d	excuse (n.)	exc u se (v.)	cloth	cl o th*

*Note vowel change.

B. Say one word in each pair below to a partner. Have your partner raise one finger if the first word was heard, and two fingers if the second was heard.

/-t/	/—d/	/-s/	/—z/
colt	c o ld	loose	lose
lent	l e nd	sauce	saws
sent	s e nd	close (adj.)	close (v.)
right	r i de	rice	rise

/-θ/	/—ð/
mouth (n.)	m ou th (v.)
sheath	sh ea the

SOUNDS IN CONTEXT: PHRASE BY PHRASE 1

Listen and underline the content words. Then rewind the tape and practice the passage in short phrases.

Tina and David Taylor, | my nextdoor neighbors, |
take good care of their home. | On Saturday, | I couldn't help noticing |
their whole family | working in the backyard. | I think |
they wanted to do | a lot of things, | because they started pretty early |
in the morning. | Tina weeded the garden | and added fertilizer |
to the vegetables. | Her daughter, | Debbie, | raked up the dead leaves |
and mowed the lawn. | Meanwhile, | David patched a hole |
in the roof of the shed. | Even little Tommy | lent a hand. |

He climbed up and down the ladder | and got the tools |
his father needed. | Later, | David made a couple of flower boxes. |
The kids planted | some tulips and daisies in them. |
Their mother picked | some corn and tomatoes |
and took them into the house. | Then she pulled out the garden hose |
and watered the whole yard. | When I looked out the window again |
in the afternoon, | they'd finished everything. |
I was so impressed | by the results of their work | that it's inspired me |
to clean up my own backyard!

SOUNDS IN CONTEXT: PHRASE BY PHRASE 2

Listen and underline the extra syllable /ɪd/ sounds. Note that not all **ed** spellings are pronounced as an extra syllable. Then rewind the tape and practice the passage in longer phrases.

Tina and David Taylor, my nextdoor neighbors, |
take good care of their home. | On Saturday, |
I couldn't help noticing their whole family working in the backyard. |
I think they want<u>ed</u> to do a lot of things, |
because they started pretty early in the morning. |
Tina weeded the garden | and added fertilizer to the vegetables. |
Her daughter, Debbie, raked up the dead leaves | and mowed the lawn.|
Meanwhile, | David patched a hole in the roof of the shed. |
Even little Tommy lent a hand. | He climbed up and down the ladder |
and got the tools his father needed. | Later, |
David made a couple of flower boxes. |
The kids planted some tulips and daisies in them. |
Their mother picked some corn and tomatoes |
and took them into the house. | Then she pulled out the garden hose |
and watered the whole yard. |
When I looked out the window again in the afternoon, |
they'd finished everything. |
I was so impressed by the results of their work |
that it's inspired me to clean up my own backyard!

SOUNDS IN CONTEXT: PHRASE BY PHRASE 3

Listen and underline the /d/ and /t/ sounds. If /t/ is pronounced with a puff of air, underline it twice. Then rewind the tape and practice the passage in complete sentences.

<u>T</u>ina and <u>D</u>avid <u>T</u>aylor, my nex<u>t</u>door neighbors, |
take goo<u>d</u> care of their home. | On Saturday, I couldn't help noticing
their whole family working in the backyard. | I guess they wanted to do

a lot of things, because they started pretty early in the morning. |
Tina weeded the garden and added fertilizer to the vegetables. |
Her daughter, Debbie, raked up the dead leaves and mowed the lawn. |
Meanwhile, David patched a hole in the roof of the shed. |
Even little Tommy lent a hand. | He climbed up and down the ladder
and got the tools his father needed. | Later, David made
a couple of flower boxes. | The kids planted some tulips and daisies
in them. | Their mother picked some corn and tomatoes and took them |
into the house. | Then she pulled out the garden hose
and watered the whole yard. | When I looked out the window again
in the afternoon, they'd finished everything. | I was so impressed
by the results of their work that it's inspired me to clean up
my own backyard! |

ON YOUR OWN

Review the **Sound Focus** exercises introduced in this lesson.
Practice the **Phrase by Phrase** steps several times.
Record the passage from beginning to end without stopping.

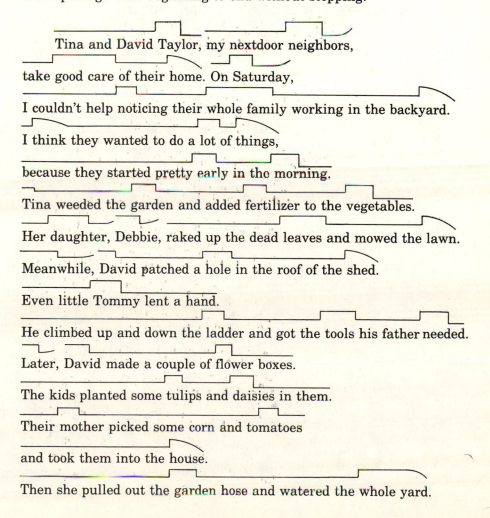

Tina and David Taylor, my nextdoor neighbors,

take good care of their home. On Saturday,

I couldn't help noticing their whole family working in the backyard.

I think they wanted to do a lot of things,

because they started pretty early in the morning.

Tina weeded the garden and added fertilizer to the vegetables.

Her daughter, Debbie, raked up the dead leaves and mowed the lawn.

Meanwhile, David patched a hole in the roof of the shed.

Even little Tommy lent a hand.

He climbed up and down the ladder and got the tools his father needed.

Later, David made a couple of flower boxes.

The kids planted some tulips and daisies in them.

Their mother picked some corn and tomatoes

and took them into the house.

Then she pulled out the garden hose and watered the whole yard.

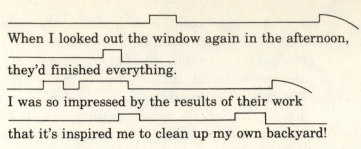

When I looked out the window again in the afternoon,

they'd finished everything.

I was so impressed by the results of their work

that it's inspired me to clean up my own backyard!

Listen to your recording.

Did you make the content words long, clear and high?
Did you make a clear difference between /t/, /d/, and /ɪd/ endings?
Did you distinguish clearly between /t/ and /d/?
Did you make a clear difference between /t/ with a puff of air and /t/ without one?
Did you lengthen vowels that come before a voiced consonant?
In which of these areas do you need to improve?
In what other areas do you need to improve?

TOPICS FOR ORAL OR WRITTEN COMPOSITION

1. Do you have a garden? What do you grow in it? Describe what you did the last time you worked in the garden.
2. Do you like to build or repair things? Tell about one of the things you made or fixed.
3. How did you spend last Saturday? Tell what you did.

Chapter 6

A Sunday Outing

VOCABULARY FOCUS

Do you or your classmates know the words in this list? Complete each sentence with a word or phrase from the list. Change nouns and verbs to appropriate forms. Discuss your choices with a partner.

break in	fishing rod	hike	swimsuit
be dying to	Frisbee	outing	talk over
east	gear	ought to	terrific
figure out	get along	pack	you bet

1. The opposite of *west* is _____.

2. To go on an _____ means to take a short pleasure trip.

3. Before going on a trip, we usually _____ our suitcases.

4. You can use a long pole called a _____ to catch fish.

5. I turned on the machine, but it wouldn't start. I can't _____ what happened to it.

6. A set of things collected together, expecially for a particular purpose, is called _____, such as camping

_____ or fishing _____.
(same word)

7. To _____ means to take a long walk through the
countryside.

8. A _____ is made especially to wear when
swimming.

9. _____ is an informal way to say "excellent."

10. My roommate and I cooperate with each other. We
_____ very well.

11. If you have a great desire to do something, you can say that you
_____ do it.

12. A _____ is a disk-shaped plaything that flies
through the air when you throw it with a spinning motion.

13. _____ is an informal phrase that means _surely_
or _I agree_.

14. Since it's very sunny, you _____ wear a hat to
protect your head.

15. Your suggestion is a good one. Let me _____ it
_____ with my coworkers.

16. I have to _____ my brand-new pair of leather
shoes; they still feel a bit stiff.

BEFORE YOU LISTEN

Look at the picture and tell what you think.

What's in the car?
Where is this family going?
What are the people in the field playing?

Dan and Jim are planning to take their families for an outing on Sunday. Dan
calls Jim up on the telephone to discuss their plans.

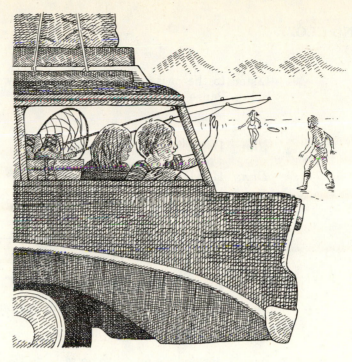

LISTENING COMPREHENSION

Read these statements. Listen to the passage and choose the best answer for each statement.

1. Jim and Dan are good friends. _____
   a. True   b. False   c. We can't tell

2. Nancy is probably Jim's _____.
   a. wife   b. daughter   c. mother

3. Pam and Dan just got home. _____
   a. True   b. False   c. We can't tell

4. Jim and Dan had not talked about going on an outing before this phone call. _____
   a. True   b. False   c. We can't tell

5. The place where they are going is called Lake _____.
   a. Hansen   b. Hansing   c. Hansom

6. Jim's children have been to this place. _____
   a. True   b. False   c. We can't tell

7. Dan _____ where the lake is.*
   a. is fairly sure b. is not sure   c. has no idea

8. Jim _____ Dan's children can swim.*
   a. is fairly sure b. is not sure   c. has no idea whether

9. Nancy's hiking boots are worn out. _____
   a. True   b. False   c. We can't tell

*Hint: listen for the intonation

LISTENING CLOZE

Listen to the passage again. Fill in the words you hear, one word for each blank. Pause the tape as necessary.

Jim: Hello?

Dan: Hi. (1) _____ is Dan.

Jim: Oh, hi, Dan. I was just going to call you.

Dan: Well, Pam and I are (2) _____ to leave the house in a minute, so I thought I (3) _____ to call you first. Have you and Nancy (4) _____ out where we're going to go for our Sunday outing?

Jim: Yeah, we (5) _____ it over with our kids and decided we ought to go to Lake Hansom. They had a lot (6) _____ fun there last time.

Dan: Lake Hansom? That's an hour and a half drive (7) _____ of here, isn't it?

Jim: Right. It's a good place to go (8) _____ and fishing. And swimming, too. Your kids can swim, (9) _____ they?

Dan: You bet! Ever (10) _____ they took lessons, they swim like fish!

Jim: Terrific! We'll all get (11) _____ just fine. Nancy's got to (12) _____ in her new hiking boots, and I'm (13) _____ to try out my new fishing rod.

Dan: Okay. We'll bring along our fishing (14) _____, swimsuits, frisbees, and stuff. Shall we take (15) _____ at eight?

Jim: I don't (16) _____. I think nine is early enough. It takes a while to get the whole family (17) _____ up and ready to go.

Dan: You're right. We'll stop by your house (18) _____ nine.

Jim: Okay. See you then.

Dan: See you later.

DISCUSSION

What other stuff might Jim's and Dan's families take with them?
Would you take along the same kind of things that they are taking?
Where do you like to go on an outing? Who usually plans the outing?

SOUND FOCUS 1: /m/

To produce the sound /m/, as in *sum*, press your lips together tightly and make a humming (voiced) sound through your nose.

Underline the letters that make the /m/ sound.

my	women	seem	sum
made	commercial	swim	room
more	chemistry	aim	home
minute	employment	time	Pam

SOUND FOCUS 2: /n/

To produce the sound /n/, as in *sun,* separate your lips and place the tip of your tongue on the upper gum ridge. Keep the sides of the tongue touching the inside of the upper teeth. Send a voiced sound through your nose.

Underline the letters that make the /n/ sound.

next	enough	Dan	own
nice	analyze	run	then
new	Nancy	thin	can't
now	invention	nine	since

SOUND FOCUS 3: /ŋ/

To produce the sound /ŋ/, as in *sung*, separate your lips and raise the back of your tongue against the back roof of the mouth. Leave the tip of your tongue relaxed behind your lower front teeth. Send a voiced sound through your nose.

Underline the letters that make the /ŋ/ sound.

along	thing	think*
hang	swing	sank
bring	wrong	finger
song	singing	language

*Note that the **n** before the sound /k/ or /g/ is pronounced /ŋ/

SOUND FOCUS 4: REDUCTIONS: *GONNA, *OUGHTA, *DUNNO

The phrases *going to, ought to,* and *don't know* are commonly reduced to **gonna,* **oughta,* and *dunno in relaxed, informal speech. The two friends in this dialog, who are speaking in a relaxed and informal manner, use these reductions. First practice the full forms. Then practice the informal forms. The asterisk (*) indicates that the phrase is a spoken (but not written) reduction.

going to leave	→ *gonna leave
going to call	→ *gonna call
ought to go	→ *oughta go
ought to see	→ *oughta see
I don't know	→ I *dunno

SOUND FOCUS 5: DIRECT ADDRESS INTONATION

When addressing a person directly by name or title, a rising intonation is usually used.

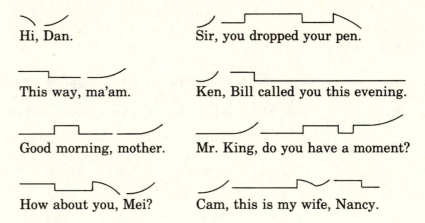

Hi, Dan.   Sir, you dropped your pen.

This way, ma'am.   Ken, Bill called you this evening.

Good morning, mother.   Mr. King, do you have a moment?

How about you, Mei?   Cam, this is my wife, Nancy.

SOUND FOCUS 6: TAG QUESTION INTONATION

A **tag question** is a short question added to the end of a statement. It can be spoken with either a rising or a falling intonation, depending on the meaning the speaker wishes to express.

A. If you (the speaker) are not quite sure whether your statement is right, and you are truly seeking information, use rising intonation as for a *Yes/No* question.

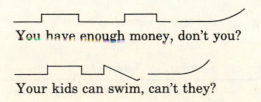

You have enough money, don't you?

Your kids can swim, can't they?

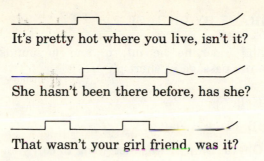

It's pretty hot where you live, isn't it?

She hasn't been there before, has she?

That wasn't your girl friend, was it?

B. If you are almost certain that your statement is right, and you are expecting the listener to agree with you, use falling intonation as for a statement.

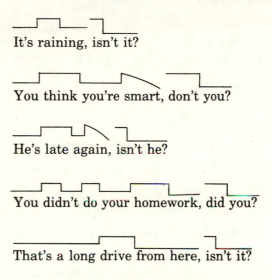

It's raining, isn't it?

You think you're smart, don't you?

He's late again, isn't he?

You didn't do your homework, did you?

That's a long drive from here, isn't it?

SOUND FOCUS 7: TWO-WORD VERB STRESS

A **two-word verb** is an idiom consisting of a verb plus a preposition or adverb. Most two-word verbs take their main stress on the second word.[1]

break ín	get alóng	grow úp
bring alóng	let gó	stand úp
clean úp	look áfter	take óff
come bý	pack úp	talk óver
figure óut	put ón	turn ón
find óut	stop bý	try óut

---

[1]Separable two-word verbs (those whose two parts may be separated by a direct object) and some inseparable two-word verbs (those whose parts may not be separated by a direct object) are stressed on the second word.

SOUNDS IN CONTEXT: PHRASE BY PHRASE 1

Listen and underline the /m/, /n/, and /ŋ/ sounds. Then rewind the tape and practice the passage in short phrases.

Jim: Hello? |

Dan: Hi. | This is Dan. |

Jim: Oh, hi, Dan. | I was just going to call you. |

Dan: Well, | Pam and I | are going to leave the house |
in a minute, | so I thought | I ought to call you first. |
Have you and Nancy figured out | where we're going to go |
for our Sunday outing? |

Jim: Yeah, | we talked it over with our kids | and decided we ought to go |
to Lake Hansom. | They had a lot of fun there | last time. |

Dan: Lake Hansom? | That's an hour and a half drive | east of here, |
isn't it? |

Jim: Right. | It's a good place | to go hiking and fishing. |
And swimming, too. | Your kids can swim, | can't they? |

Dan: You bet! | Ever since they took lessons, | they swim like fish! |

Jim: Terrific! | We'll all get along just fine. | Nancy's got to break in |
her new hiking boots, | and I'm dying to try out |
my new fishing rod. |

Dan: Okay. | We'll bring along our fishing gear, | swimsuits, | frisbees, |
and stuff. | Shall we take off at eight? |

Jim: I don't know. | I think nine is early enough. | It takes a while |
to get the whole family packed up | and ready to go. |

Dan: You're right. | We'll stop by your house at nine. |

Jim: Okay. | See you then. |

Dan: See you later.

SOUNDS IN CONTEXT: PHRASE BY PHRASE 2

Listen and underline the contractions and reductions. Circle the direct addresses and tag questions. Then rewind the tape and practice the passage in complete sentences.

Jim: Hello? |

Dan: Hi. This is Dan. |

Jim: Oh, hi, (Dan) | I was just going to call you. |

Dan: Well, Pam and I are going to leave the house in a minute,

so I thought I ought to call you first. | Have you and Nancy

figured out where we're going to go for our Sunday outing? |

Jim: Yeah, we talked it over with our kids and decided we ought to go

to Lake Hansom. | They had a lot of fun there last time. |

Dan: Lake Hansom? | That's an hour and a half drive east of here,

isn't it? |

Jim: Right. | It's a good place to go hiking and fishing. |

And swimming, too. | Your kids can swim, can't they? |

Dan: You bet! | Ever since they took lessons, they swim like fish! |

Jim: Terrific! | We'll all get along just fine. |

Nancy's got to break in her new hiking boots,

and I'm dying to try out my new fishing rod. |

Dan: Okay. | We'll bring along our fishing gear, swimsuits, frisbees,

and stuff. | Shall we take off at eight? |

Jim: I don't know. | I think nine is early enough. | It takes a while

to get the whole family packed up and ready to go. |

Dan: You're right. | We'll stop by your house at nine. |

Jim: Okay. | See you then. |

Dan: See you later.

ON YOUR OWN

Review the **Sound Focus** exercises introduced in this lesson.
Practice **Phrase by Phrase 1** and **2** several times.
Record the passage from beginning to end without stopping.

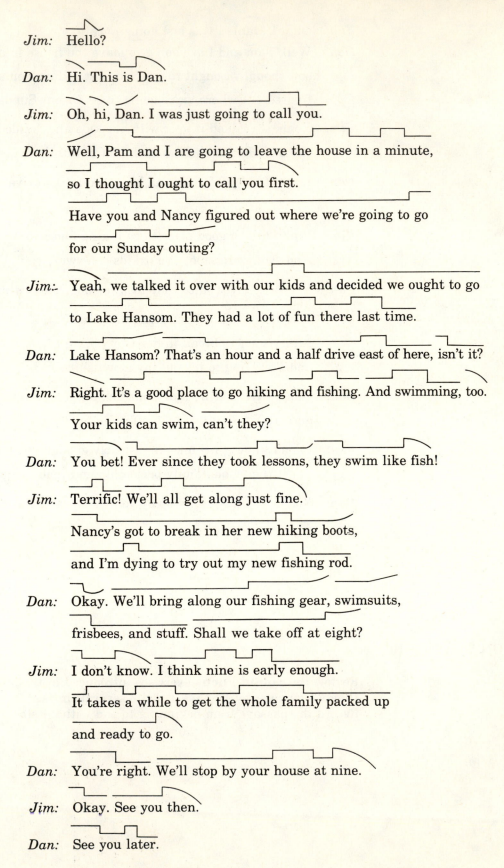

Jim: Hello?

Dan: Hi. This is Dan.

Jim: Oh, hi, Dan. I was just going to call you.

Dan: Well, Pam and I are going to leave the house in a minute,

so I thought I ought to call you first.

Have you and Nancy figured out where we're going to go

for our Sunday outing?

Jim: Yeah, we talked it over with our kids and decided we ought to go

to Lake Hansom. They had a lot of fun there last time.

Dan: Lake Hansom? That's an hour and a half drive east of here, isn't it?

Jim: Right. It's a good place to go hiking and fishing. And swimming, too.
Your kids can swim, can't they?

Dan: You bet! Ever since they took lessons, they swim like fish!

Jim: Terrific! We'll all get along just fine.

Nancy's got to break in her new hiking boots,

and I'm dying to try out my new fishing rod.

Dan: Okay. We'll bring along our fishing gear, swimsuits,

frisbees, and stuff. Shall we take off at eight?

Jim: I don't know. I think nine is early enough.

It takes a while to get the whole family packed up

and ready to go.

Dan: You're right. We'll stop by your house at nine.

Jim: Okay. See you then.

Dan: See you later.

Listen to your recording.

Did you pronounce the sounds /m/, /n/ and /ŋ/ clearly?

Did you reduce the phrase "going to" to "*gonna," "ought to" to "*oughta" and "don't know" to "*dunno"?

Did you distinguish between rising intonation and falling intonation?

In which of these areas do you need to improve?

In what other areas do you need to improve?

TOPICS FOR ORAL OR WRITTEN COMPOSITION

1. Describe an outing that you took. Tell when and where you went, who went with you, how you passed the time, and any unusual incident that may have happened.

2. Describe the process involved in planning an outing. What do you need to think about before going out? What are the steps you need to take before the plans are set?

Chapter 7

The Oak and the Reed

VOCABULARY FOCUS

Do you or your classmates know the *italicized* words in the following sentences? Match each word with a synonym from the list below. Write the letter in the blank. Discuss your choices with a partner.

1. _____ There is a tall *oak* growing behind our house.

2. _____ *Reeds* grow in wet places.

3. _____ This thick paper is *firm* enough to make a sign that won't bend.

4. _____ The *boughs* of the trees were heavy with hundreds of apples.

5. _____ The child *stooped* to pick up a pretty shell on the beach.

6. _____ On a hot day, a *breeze* feels very refreshing.

7. _____ When the storm came, the sky was filled with *lightning* and thunder.

8. _____ The wheat *swayed* as the wind blew back and forth.

9. _____ Mr. Tony died young. It was alcohol that caused his *ruin*.

10. _____ While I was fishing, I lost my balance and *toppled* into the lake.

11. _____ The *rim* of a cup is bigger than the *rim* of a bottle.

12. _____ The tree was struck down by a *mighty* wind.

13. _____ At the end of his performance, the singer *bowed* to the audience.

14. _____ When the bank was robbed, the police questioned several people who were seen running from the bank.

15. _____ Dean's average in the class is 95% and Joe's average is 78%. Dean's grades are *superior to* Joe's.

16. _____ When our professor is lecturing in front of the class, he acts in a *dignified* manner. When he is among his close friends, he behaves in a more informal and relaxed manner.

17. _____ Although Peter is very clever, he does not try to make other people think he is important. He acts in a *humble* manner.

18. _____ When Mona lost her job, her friends offered her some money. She thanked them, but she wouldn't accept their money because of her *pride*.

A. asked with doubt	G. gentle wind	M. main branches
B. bent down	H. grasslike plants	N. modest
C. bent forward	I. great	O. formal or noble
D. fell	J. a hardwood tree	P. self-respect
E. destruction	K. higher than	Q. stiff
F. edge	L. light from the sky	R. swung

BEFORE YOU LISTEN

Look at the picture and tell what you think.

Where are the oak and the reed growing?
Describe their expressions.
What's the weather like?

This is another fable by Aesop. It cautions people not to act too proudly.

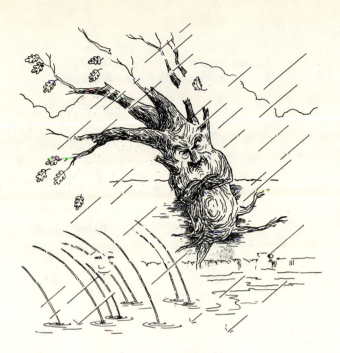

LISTENING COMPREHENSION

Read these statements. Listen to the passage and choose the best answer for each statement.

1. The oak tree and the reed _____ spoke to each other.
   a. never
   b. rarely
   c. sometimes
   d. usually

2. Which is true? _____
   a. The oak looked up to the reed.
   b. The reed looked up to the oak.
   c. The oak looked down on the reed.
   d. The reed looked down on the oak.

3. Compared to the reed, the oak was _____.
   a. stronger
   b. more dignified
   c. prouder
   d. smarter

4. The oak was destroyed by _____.
   a. the reed
   b. the river
   c. a flash of lightning
   d. the wind

5. The reed was _____ than the oak.
   a. kinder
   b. higher
   c. more flexible
   d. more powerful

6. The moral of this fable is _____.
   a. Be proud and firm.
   b. Be shy and passive.
   c. Be kind to your neighbors.
   d. Be humble and flexible.

LISTENING CLOZE

Listen to the passage again. Fill in the words you hear, one word for each blank. Pause the tape as necessary.

An oak tree and a reed (1) _____ side by side

on the rim of a river. From time to time they spoke to

(2) _____ other, but they weren't

(3) _____ friends. The mighty oak thought he was

far (4) _____ to the humble reed and,

from a great height, looked down on him.

"Don't you have any (5) _____?" the oak

questioned the reed. "You bend and (6) _____ to

the lightest (7) _____. You ought to be more

dignified. You (8) _____ to stand up straight the

way I do. No wind can make me (9) _____ or lower

myself."

Just as he spoke an (10) _____ storm began.

Lightning flashed and a strong wind shook the trees. The oak

(11) _____ the storm, standing

(12) _____ for a short while. But his very stiffness

caused his (13) _____.

The wind struck hard against him, (14) _____

his branches, broke his biggest (15) _____, and

toppled him into the river. But the reed (16) _____

and bent, letting the wind blow over him. And when the storm

(17) _____, he was still growing

(18) _____ the rim of the river.

DISCUSSION

What value does this fable have in modern life?
Is there a fable like this one in your language?
Do you think you are more like an oak or a reed?

SOUND FOCUS 1: /iʸ/

To produce the sound /iʸ/, as in _reed_, raise your tongue high in your mouth and make the muscles of your tongue and cheeks tense. Pull the edges of your mouth outward and make a voiced sound.

Underline the letters that make the sound /iʸ/.

be	reed	cheese[1]
key	brief	machine
see	clean	sleepy
tree	breeze	receive

SOUND FOCUS 2: /ɪ/

To produce the sound /ɪ/, as in *river*, raise your tongue high in your mouth (but not as high as for /iʸ/). Keep the muscles of your tongue, lips and cheeks relaxed and make a voiced sound.

Underline the letters that make the sound /ɪ/.

rim	river	himself
him	biggest	insisting
wind	stiffness	consider
his	into	dignified

SOUND FOCUS 3: /oʷ/

To produce the sound /oʷ/, as in *oak*, round your lips, letting the back of your tongue and your jaw move from a low to a mid position. As you move your tongue and jaw, make your lips become more rounded. This produces a gliding sound. Make a voiced sound.

Underline the letters that make the sound /oʷ/.

no	oak	over
show	coat	open
toe	don't	growing
blow	close	although

SOUND FOCUS 4: /ɔ/

To produce the sound /ɔ/, as in *saw*, round the lips slightly (less than for /oʷ/), lower your jaw (more than for /oʷ/) and place the back of your tongue in a low position. Make a voiced sound. Do not change the roundness of your lips or

---

[1]*When taking a photograph, a photographer often tells the people in the photograph to say "cheese" in order to make them smile with the sound /iʸ/.

move your jaw; /ɔ/ is not a gliding vowel. Underline the letters that make the sound /ɔ/.

s<u>aw</u>	fought	cough
cause	taught	strong
call	thought	awful
ought	walk	always

SOUND FOCUS 5: CONTRAST /iʸ/-/ɪ/, /oʷ/-/ɔ/

A. First listen to each pair of words to hear the difference between them. Then practice saying them, distinguishing clearly between /iʸ/ and /ɪ/.

beat - bit	leap - lip	green - grin
seat - sit	cheap - chip	leave - live
reed - rid	peach - pitch	ream - rim

B. First listen to each pair of words to hear the difference between them. Then practice saying them, distinguishing clearly between /oʷ/ and /ɔ/.

low - law	coal - call	boat - bought
loan - lawn	owed - awed	woke - walk
pose - pause	oat - ought	coat - caught

SOUNDS IN CONTEXT: PHRASE BY PHRASE 1

Listen and underline the content words. Notice that these words are longer and clearer than the function words. Also find one function word that is stressed for contrast. Then rewind the tape and practice the passage in short phrases. While you speak, clap out the content words.

An <u>oak</u> <u>tree</u> and a <u>reed</u> | <u>grew</u> <u>side</u> by <u>side</u> | on the <u>rim</u> of a <u>river.</u> |
From time to time | they spoke to each other, |
but they weren't close friends. | The mighty oak |
thought he was far superior | to the humble reed | and, |
from a great height, | looked down on him. |
"Don't you have any pride?" | the oak questioned the reed. |
"You bend and bow | to the lightest breeze. |
You ought to be more dignified. | You ought to stand up straight |
the way I do. | No wind can make me | stoop or lower myself." |
Just as he spoke | an awful storm began. | Lightning flashed |
and a strong wind | shook the trees. | The oak fought the storm, |

standing firm | for a short while. | But his very stiffness |
caused his ruin. |

    The wind struck hard against him, | tore his branches, |
broke his biggest boughs, | and toppled him | into the river. |
But the reed swayed and bent, | letting the wind blow over him. |
And when the storm passed, | he was still growing |
on the rim of the river. |

SOUNDS IN CONTEXT: PHRASE BY PHRASE 2

Listen and underline the /i^y/ sounds once and the /ɪ/ sounds twice. (Note that
/ɪ/ sounds can be written with i, and /i^y/ sounds with **e, ee, ea, ei, ey, i, ie, y,**
and **ey.**) Then rewind the tape and practice the passage in longer phrases.

    An oak tree and a reed | grew side by side on the rim of a river. |
From time to time they spoke to each other, |
but they weren't close friends. |
The mighty oak thought he was far superior | to the humble reed |
and, from a great height, | looked down on him. |

    "Don't you have any pride?" | the oak questioned the reed. |
"You bend and bow | to the lightest breeze. |
You ought to be more dignified. | You ought to stand up straight |
the way I do. | No wind can make me stoop or lower myself."

    Just as he spoke | an awful storm began. | Lightning flashed |
and a strong wind shook the trees. | The oak fought the storm, |
standing firm for a short while. |
But his very stiffness caused his ruin. |

    The wind struck hard against him, |
tore his branches, broke his biggest boughs, |
and toppled him into the river. | But the reed swayed and bent, |
letting the wind blow over him. | And when the storm passed, |
he was still growing on the rim of the river. |

SOUNDS IN CONTEXT: PHRASE BY PHRASE 3

Listen and underline the /ɔ/ sounds once and the /o^w/ sounds twice. (Note that
/ɔ/ sounds can be written with **o, ou, au, aw, a,** and **al,** and /o^w/ sounds with **o,
ou, ow, oe,** and **oa.**) Then rewind the tape and practice the passage in complete sentences.

    An oak tree and a reed grew side by side on the rim of a river. |
From time to time they spoke to each other, but they weren't close
friends. | The mighty oak thought he was far superior
to the humble reed and, from a great height, looked down on him. |

    "Don't you have any pride?" the oak questioned the reed. |
"You bend and bow to the lightest breeze. | You ought to be more

dignified. | You ought to stand up straight the way I do. |
No wind can make me stoop or lower myself."

Just as he spoke an awful storm began. |
Lightning flashed and a strong wind shook the trees. |
The oak fought the storm, standing firm for a short while. |
But his very stiffness caused his ruin. |

The wind struck hard against him, tore his branches,
broke his biggest boughs, and toppled him into the river. |
But the reed swayed and bent, letting the wind blow over him. |
And when the storm passed, he was still growing
on the rim of the river. |

ON YOUR OWN

Review the **Sound Focus** exercises introduced in this lesson.
Practice the **Phrase by Phrase** steps several times.
Record the passage from beginning to end without stopping.

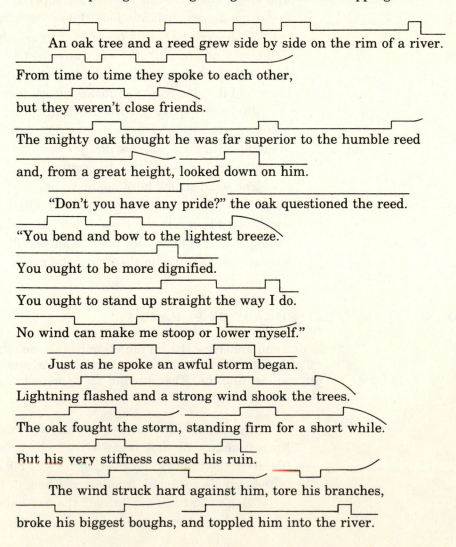

An oak tree and a reed grew side by side on the rim of a river.

From time to time they spoke to each other,

but they weren't close friends.

The mighty oak thought he was far superior to the humble reed

and, from a great height, looked down on him.

"Don't you have any pride?" the oak questioned the reed.

"You bend and bow to the lightest breeze.

You ought to be more dignified.

You ought to stand up straight the way I do.

No wind can make me stoop or lower myself."

Just as he spoke an awful storm began.

Lightning flashed and a strong wind shook the trees.

The oak fought the storm, standing firm for a short while.

But his very stiffness caused his ruin.

The wind struck hard against him, tore his branches,

broke his biggest boughs, and toppled him into the river.

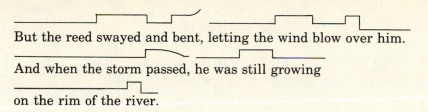

But the reed swayed and bent, letting the wind blow over him.

And when the storm passed, he was still growing

on the rim of the river.

Listen to your recording.

Did you make the content words longer and clearer than the function words? Did you stress the pronoun "I" for contrast?
Did you make a clear difference between the sounds /iʸ/ and /ɪ/?
Did you make a clear difference between the sounds /oʷ/ and /ɔ/?

TOPICS FOR ORAL OR WRITTEN COMPOSITION

1. Describe a real-life situation which reflects the moral of "The Oak and the Reed."
2. Point out the natural characteristics of an oak tree and a reed. Explain why they were used in this fable to represent a proud person and a humble person. What other pair of plants could be used to tell a fable with the same moral?

Chapter 8

Koko's Kitten

VOCABULARY FOCUS

Do you or your classmates know the words in this list? Complete each sentence with a word or phrase from the list. Change nouns and verbs to appropriate forms. Discuss your choices with a partner.

cheek	consist	kiss	take a liking to
comfort	converse	kitten	treat
communicate	gorilla	napkin	vocabulary
compound	hug	sign language	whiskers

1. A _____ is a strong animal that looks like a large monkey without a tail.

2. A young cat is called a _____.

3. The long stiff hairs that grow near an animal's mouth are called _____.

4. The _____ is the soft part of the face below each eye.

5. If I get food on my mouth and hands during a meal, I wipe it off with a _____.

6. The mother picked up her baby and _____ him gently on the cheek.

7. Then she took him in her arms and _____ him tightly.

8. I'd rather relax in the _____ of my own home than in a stranger's home.

9. The more words I learn, the bigger my _____ grows.

10. By raising his hand, the student _____ to the teacher that he wanted to ask a question.

11. As my pronunciation and listening skills improve, it gets easier for me to _____ with English speakers.

12. Many deaf people use _____ to exchange ideas.

13. Mack likes his boss because she _____ all her employees very kindly.

14. Cathy didn't like milk when she first tasted it, but after a while she _____ to it.

15. Gary's office is not in this group of buildings. It's located in the _____ across the street.

16. The United States of America _____ of 50 states plus the District of Columbia.

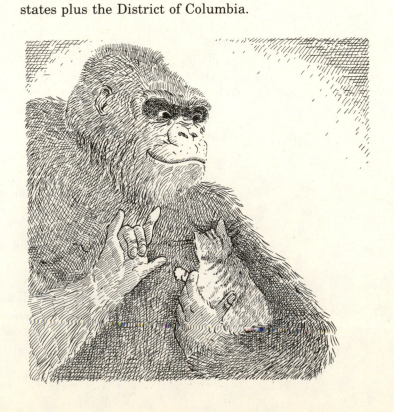

BEFORE YOU LISTEN

Look at the picture and tell what you think.

Does the gorilla look happy? angry? sad? puzzled? surprised?
How do you think the kitten feels?
Can the gorilla talk to the kitten?[1]

Koko is a gorilla that lives at the Gorilla Foundation of California. Dr. Francine Patterson and her fellow researchers study how Koko and other gorillas learn to understand and use language. In this passage, you will find out how Koko fell in love with a kitten.

LISTENING COMPREHENSION

Read these statements. Listen to the passage and choose the best answer for each statement.

1. Koko is a _____ -year-old gorilla.
   a. three
   b. thirteen
   c. thirty
   d. thirty-three

2. American Sign Language is used by _____.
   a. most animals
   b. gorillas and cats
   c. people who can't hear well
   d. people who can't speak English

3. Koko can understand _____ signs in American Sign Language.
   a. 500
   b. 1,000
   c. 9,000
   d. 10,000

4. To show that she wanted a cat, Koko _____.
   a. pulled her whiskers
   b. pulled her cheeks
   c. pulled a cat's whiskers
   d. pulled her fingers across her face

5. When Koko saw the kittens, she _____ that she loved them.
   a. signed
   b. sighed
   c. said
   d. saw

6. Koko took a special liking to the kitten that had no _____.
   a. mother
   b. name
   c. whiskers
   d. tail

7. Koko _____ All Ball.
   a. kissed
   b. carried
   c. hugged
   d. all of the above

8. Koko gave All Ball napkins _____.
   a. to wipe his mouth
   b. to keep his body clean
   c. to wear as clothes
   d. to play games with

_____

[1]The gorilla is signing "I love you" in American Sign Language.

LISTENING CLOZE

Listen to the passage again. Fill in the words you hear, one word for each blank. Pause the tape as necessary.

Can a tiny cat and a big gorilla find (1) _____

together? Well, you can ask Koko this question. Koko is a thirteen-

(2) _____ -old gorilla who

(3) _____ in American Sign Language, the hand

language of (4) _____ people. Koko's vocabulary

(5) _____ of over one thousand signs in this

language. By pulling two (6) _____ across her

cheeks, like (7) _____, Koko communicated that

she wanted a cat. One day, three kittens were taken as

(8) _____ to the gorilla compound where Koko

lives. When Koko saw the (9) _____, she got very

excited and (10) _____ that she loved them. She

took a special (11) _____ to the one that

(12) _____ no tail. She picked this kitten up and

(13) _____ him the name All Ball. Koko

(14) _____ the kitten as if he were a baby gorilla.

She carried him in her arms, and

(15) _____ and kissed him. She gave him

(16) _____ to wear as clothes, and played

(17) _____ with him. I'd guess All Ball was

(18) _____ to get such love and attention. Wouldn't

you?

DISCUSSION

Is it possible to fall in love at first sight?
How do you think All Ball felt about Koko?
Do you think gorillas are more intelligent than other animals?

SOUND FOCUS 1: /k/

A. To produce the sound /k/, as in _cat,_ open your mouth slightly and press the back of your tongue against the back roof of your mouth. This stops the air from flowing out of your mouth. When the sound /k/ comes before a vowel in a stressed syllable, release a sharp, strong, voiceless puff of air as you pull the back of your tongue away from the roof of your mouth.[2]

Underline the letters that make the sound /k/.

c̲at	can't	record (verb)
kittens	comfort	occur
kissed	compound	mechanic
carried	question	vocabulary

B. When the sound /k/ comes at the end of a phrase, do not let your tongue break contact with the roof of your mouth. When the sound /k/ comes at the beginning of an unstressed syllable, or after the sound /s/, do not release a puff of air.[3]

ma̲ke	orchestra	record (noun)
took	consist	Koko[4]
picked	liking	scrape
technique	napkins	whiskers

SOUND FOCUS 2: /g/

To produce the sound /g/, as in *get*, open your mouth slightly and press the back of your tongue against the back roof of your mouth, as for the sound /k/. Then let your tongue break contact while you make a voiced sound. Do not release a puff of air. Like other stop consonants, /g/ is not released at the end of a word.

Underline the letters that make the sound /g/.

g̲et	go	fingers	big
guess	good	language	leg
games	gorilla	grass	flag
gave	together	glad	hug

SOUND FOCUS 3: VOWEL LENGTH

A. The first word in each pair below ends in a voiceless /k/. The second word ends in a voiced /g/. Hold the vowel longer when it is followed by the voiced /g/.

---

[2]Test yourself by placing your hand in front of your mouth and feeling a puff of air. If you hold up a small piece of paper, it should move suddenly as you pronounce the sound /k/.

[3]Test yourself by looking at your tongue in a mirror and by placing your hand in front of your mouth.

[4]Release a puff of air on the first /k/ but not on the second.

/-k/	/—g/
Huck	h u g
duck	d u g
pick	p i g
back	b a g

B. Underline the long vowels in the following sentences. Then practice saying them, paying attention to vowel length.

Huck hugged the duck.

Peg picked the dog.

Did Pat like the plays?

This place is ice cold.

Jack rode a colt.

Did Liz breathe deeply?

She took a big breath.

SOUND FOCUS 4: PHRASE STRESS

A. Compared to function words, content words are longer, clearer, stronger and sometimes higher in pitch.

Look at my stomach!

The most important word, or **key word,** of the phrase receives the most emphasis. The rising or falling intonation is emphasized on the stressed syllable of this key word.

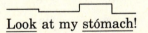

Look at my stómach!

Usually the key word is the last content word in a phrase.

Please speak loúdly.

Let's eat at hóme.

I was just going to cáll you.

He bought a new cóat.

I took ten dóllars with me.

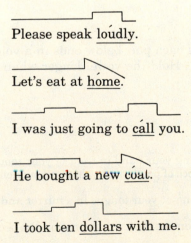

B. Phrase stress is determined by context. It depends on what the speaker considers most important. When a new idea is introduced, the new idea is emphasized and the old idea is not.

Please speak loudly. But not too loudly.

Let's eat at home. At your home.

I was just going to call you. Or, at least, try to call you.

He bought a new coat. He gave the old coat away.

C. Underline the key words. If the key word has more than one syllable, mark the stressed syllable.

I can play the piano. I can play ten songs on the piano.

{ Can Koko and All Ball find comfort together?

  Yes, comfort and happiness.

I'm dying to try out my new fishing rod since I broke my old one.

SOUND FOCUS 5: NOUN COMPOUNDS

A. A **noun compound** is composed of two words that function as a single noun. The main stress is on the first word of the compound.[5] Compare the stress and intonation of these phrases.

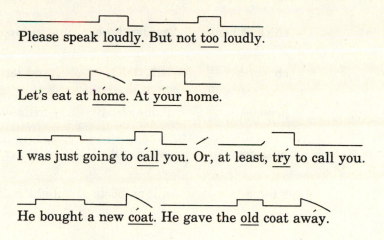

Adjective + Noun	Noun Compound
good teacher	English teacher
long board	blackboard
baby sister	baby sitter

[5]Noun + Noun and Adj. + Noun are the most common combinations.

B. Practice saying these noun compounds to a partner.

grásshopper	náme-calling	físhing gear
chicken bones	garden hose	sign language
chopsticks	oak tree	hand language
headache	fishing rod	gorilla compound
push-ups	swim suit	teenager
sit-ups	hiking boots	light bulb

SOUNDS IN CONTEXT: PHRASE BY PHRASE 1:

Listen and mark (with ´) the key word(s) in each phrase. Then rewind the tape and practice the passage in short phrases.

Can a tiny cát | and a big gorílla | find cómfort together? | Well, | you can ask Koko this question. | Koko is a thirteen-year-old gorilla | who converses in American Sign Language, | the hand language | of deaf people. | Koko's vocabulary | consists of over one thousand signs | in this language. | By pulling two fingers across her cheeks, | like whiskers, | Koko communicated | that she wanted a cat. | One day, | three kittens were taken as gifts | to the gorilla compound | where Koko lives. | When Koko saw the kittens, | she got very excited | and signed that she loved them. | She took a special liking | to the one that had no tail. | She picked this kitten up | and gave him the name | All Ball. | Koko treated the kitten | as if he were a baby gorilla. | She carried him in her arms, | and hugged and kissed him. | She gave him napkins | to wear as clothes, | and played games with him. | I'd guess All Ball was glad | to get such love and attention. | Wouldn't you? |

SOUNDS IN CONTEXT: PHRASE BY PHRASE 2:

Listen and underline the /k/ sounds. If the /k/ sound is pronounced with a puff of air, underline it twice. (Note that /k/ sounds can be written with **k, c** and **qu.**)

<u><u>K</u></u>o<u>k</u>o's <u><u>K</u></u>itten

Then rewind the tape and practice the passage in longer phrases.

Can a tiny cat and a big gorilla | find comfort together? | Well, |
you can ask Koko this question. | Koko is a thirteen-year-old gorilla |
who converses in American Sign Language, |
the hand language of deaf people. | Koko's vocabulary |
consists of over one thousand signs | in this language. |
By pulling two fingers across her cheeks, | like whiskers, |
Koko communicated that she wanted a cat. |
One day, three kittens were taken as gifts |
to the gorilla compound where Koko lives. |
When Koko saw the kittens, |
she got very excited and signed that she loved them. |
She took a special liking to the one that had no tail. |
She picked this kitten up | and gave him the name All Ball. |
Koko treated the kitten | as if he were a baby gorilla. |
She carried him in her arms, | and hugged and kissed him. |
She gave him napkins to wear as clothes, |
and played games with him. |
I'd guess All Ball was glad |
to get such love and attention. |
Wouldn't you? |

SOUNDS IN CONTEXT: PHRASE BY PHRASE 3:

Listen and underline the /g/ sounds. Note that some, but not all, **g** spellings are pronounced /g/.

sign lan<u>g</u>uage

Then rewind the tape and practice the passage in complete sentences.

Can a tiny cat and a big gorilla find comfort together? |

Well, you can ask Koko this question. | Koko is a thirteen-year-old

gorilla who converses in American Sign Language, the hand language

of deaf people. | Koko's vocabulary consists of over one thousand signs

in this language. | By pulling two fingers across her cheeks, like whiskers, Koko communicated that she wanted a cat. | One day,

three kittens were taken as gifts to the gorilla compound

where Koko lives. | When Koko saw the kittens, she got very excited

and signed that she loved them. | She took a special liking to the one

that had no tail. | She picked this kitten up

and gave him the name All Ball. | Koko treated the kitten

as if he were a baby gorilla. | She carried him in her arms,

and hugged and kissed him. | She gave him napkins to wear as clothes,

and played games with him. | I'd guess All Ball was glad

to get such love and attention. | Wouldn't you? |

ON YOUR OWN

Review the **Sound Focus** exercises introduced in this lesson.
Practice the **Phrase by Phrase** steps several times.
Record the passage from beginning to end without stopping.

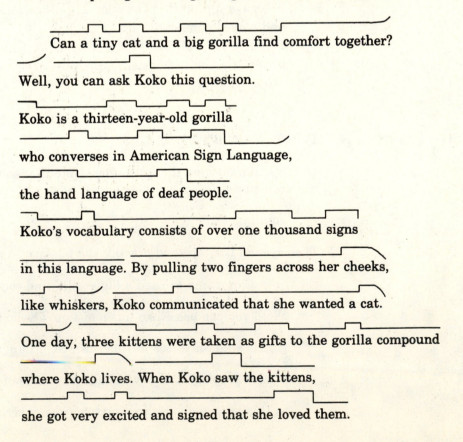

Can a tiny cat and a big gorilla find comfort together?

Well, you can ask Koko this question.

Koko is a thirteen-year-old gorilla

who converses in American Sign Language,

the hand language of deaf people.

Koko's vocabulary consists of over one thousand signs

in this language. By pulling two fingers across her cheeks,

like whiskers, Koko communicated that she wanted a cat.

One day, three kittens were taken as gifts to the gorilla compound

where Koko lives. When Koko saw the kittens,

she got very excited and signed that she loved them.

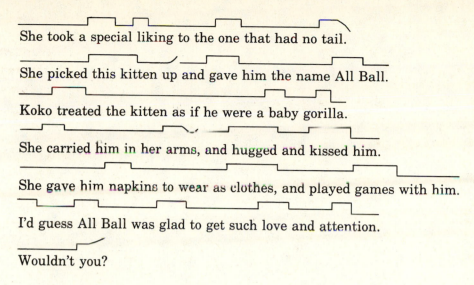

She took a special liking to the one that had no tail.

She picked this kitten up and gave him the name All Ball.

Koko treated the kitten as if he were a baby gorilla.

She carried him in her arms, and hugged and kissed him.

She gave him napkins to wear as clothes, and played games with him.

I'd guess All Ball was glad to get such love and attention.

Wouldn't you?

Listen to your recording.

Did you stress the key words in each phrase?

Did you make the content words longer and clearer than the function words?

Did you stress the first word of noun compounds?

Did you pronounce the sounds /k/ and /g/ clearly?

Did you make a clear difference between /k/ with a puff of air and /k/ without one?

In which of these areas do you need to improve?

In what other areas do you need to improve?

TOPICS FOR ORAL OR WRITTEN COMPOSITION

1. How much can a human being teach an animal? Choose one animal, such as a dog, a chimpanzee, a gorilla, or a horse, and tell what it can learn. Base your ideas on what has been accomplished scientifically or from your own experience with that kind of animal.

2. Describe how a particular kind of animal communicates with human beings. What actions and sounds does it use to show what it wants, what it likes, how it feels?

3. What problems does a deaf and/or mute person (one who is unable to speak) encounter? How important is sign language to a deaf or mute person?

Chapter 9

Why I Work

VOCABULARY FOCUS

Do you or your classmates know the following *italicized* words? Two of the three words or phrases afterward are synonyms. One is not a synonym. Cross out the one that is not a synonym. Discuss your choices with a partner.

1. *accomplish:*   a. achieve   b. ~~fail~~   c. complete
2. *article:*   a. essay   b. speech   c. paper
3. *complex:*   a. complicated   b. difficult   c. simple
4. *concern:*   a. care   b. neglect   c. attention
5. *constant:*   a. continual   b. nonstop   c. irregular
6. *encouragement:*   a. help   b. restriction   c. hope
7. *further:*   a. help to succeed   b. develop   c. prevent
8. *make a mark:*   a. gain success   b. gain fame   c. gain weight
9. *model:*   a. pattern   b. good example   c. shame
10. *provide:*   a. supply   b. take   c. give
11. *publish:*   a. read and write   b. write and sell   c. print and distribute
12. *purpose:*   a. aim   b. goal   c. beginning
13. *research:*   a. leisure   b. study   c. investigation
14. *reward:*   a. prize   b. fine   c. bonus
15. *satisfaction:*   a. hopelessness   b. pleasure   c. gladness
16. *serve:*   a. benefit   b. give aid to   c. trouble
17. *society:*   a. the public   b. the individual   c. the people
18. *support:*   a. take care of   b. suffer   c. pay for
19. *urge:*   a. refuse   b. advise   c. push
20. *viewpoint:*   a. point of view   b. attitude   c. action

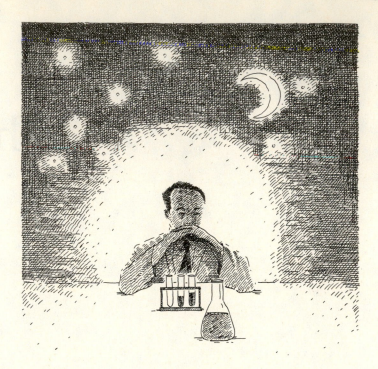

BEFORE YOU LISTEN

Look at the picture and tell what you think.

What kind of objects are on the table?
What is the man thinking about?
What's his occupation?

Wei Wang, who lives in the People's Republic of China, is involved in scientific and cultural exchange with people from the United States. He has had a chance to exchange ideas with Americans on many subjects besides his research. Here, he gives his views on working.

LISTENING COMPREHENSION

Read these statements. Listen to the passage and choose the best answer for each statement.

1. Somebody asked Wei Wang _____.
    a. where he worked
    b. why he worked
    c. how he worked.
    d. when he worked.

2. Wei Wang implies, but does not say directly, that _____.
    a. we work to serve society
    b. we work for personal satisfaction
    c. most people have nothing better to do than work
    d. people work for many reasons

3. Wei Wang's mother wanted him _____.
    a. to become a successful scientist
    b. to support her in her old age
    c. to take care of his brothers and sisters
    d. to leave a mark on society

4. Wei Wang is thankful for his mother's _____.
    a. concern
    b. encouragement
    c. support
    d. all of the above

5. Wei Wang has _____.
    a. three daughters and three sons
    b. three brothers and three sisters
    c. two brothers and three sisters
    d. two sons and three daughters

6. Wei Wang wants to _____.
    a. live only once
    b. spend his whole life supporting his children
    c. be a good model for his daughter
    d. do all of the above

LISTENING CLOZE

Listen to the passage again. Fill in the words you hear, one word for each blank. Pause the tape as necessary.

"Why do you work?" you (1) _____ me. What a complex question! Do we work to (2) _____ society or to gain personal satisfaction? Do we work to earn (3) _____ or because (4) _____ nothing better to do? Perhaps no one can (5) _____ this very well. I'll just try to (6) _____ on why I work.

When I was a child, my mother (7) _____ me to further my education. She said, "Son, you (8) _____ study hard. You have to become a famous scientist someday. That'll be my (9) _____." My mother spent her whole life supporting her children. With three sons and three daughters, she had to work very hard. (10) _____ never forget her constant concern and (11) _____. A person lives only once. I think if I haven't done something important before I (12) _____, I'll certainly be sorry! So I want to (13) _____ as much as possible. If I can make a small mark, I'll feel very happy. (14) _____ mean that my life has purpose. I've already reached a little success (15) _____ my work and published (16) _____ articles on my research. But I still want to do (17) _____ more. As a father, I want to (18) _____ a good model for my daughter.

What's your viewpoint?

DISCUSSION

Do you work for the same reasons as Wei Wang?
How does Wei Wang want to make a mark?
What are some other ways to make one's mark?
In what ways can Wei Wang provide a good model for his daughter?

SOUND FOCUS 1: /ɑ/

To produce the sound /ɑ/, as in _father_ or t<u>o</u>p, lower your jaw, relax your lips, and let the front of your tongue rest behind the lower front teeth. Make a voiced sound.

Underline the letters that make the sound /ɑ/. Draw a slash through the reduced, or _schwa_, vowels.

f<u>a</u>th/er	w<u>a</u>nt	c<u>o</u>nstant	d<u>o</u>cument
st<u>o</u>p	m<u>o</u>del	sch<u>o</u>lar	p<u>o</u>ssible
r<u>o</u>b	c<u>o</u>mment	c<u>o</u>mplex	acc<u>o</u>mplish

SOUND FOCUS 2: /ʌ/

To produce the sound /ʌ/, as in _cut,_ open your jaw somewhat less than for /a/, relax your lips, and let your tongue lie at rest in a neutral central position. Make a voiced sound.

Underline the letters that make the sound /ʌ/. Draw a slash through the reduced, or _schwa_, vowels.

c<u>u</u>t	d<u>o</u>ne	n<u>u</u>mber	bec<u>o</u>me
m<u>u</u>ch	s<u>o</u>n	m<u>o</u>ther	s<u>o</u>mething
r<u>o</u>ugh	l<u>o</u>ve	st<u>u</u>dy	p<u>u</u>blish

SOUND FOCUS 3: /ɚ/

To produce the sound /ɚ/, as in _earn_, open your jaw only slightly, pull your tongue up high, close to the center of the hard roof of the mouth, and round your lips slightly.[1] Make a voiced sound. Note that in words with the /ɚ/ sound, the vowel letter combines with the _r_ to form _one_ single sound. The sound /ɚ/ in the words in the first three columns are stressed; those in the fourth column are unstressed.

Underline the letters that make the sound /ɚ/.

<u>ear</u>n	<u>ur</u>ge	f<u>ur</u>ther	sug<u>ar</u>
s<u>er</u>ve	p<u>ur</u>pose	p<u>er</u>sonal	moth<u>er</u>
w<u>or</u>k	conc<u>er</u>n	c<u>er</u>tainly	perh<u>a</u>ps
b<u>ir</u>d	ref<u>er</u>	enc<u>our</u>age[2]	forg<u>e</u>t

---

[1]The sound /ɚ/ may be made in two ways with the same result. Some speakers curl the tip of the tongue upward, while others pull the middle of the tongue into a bunched position.
[2]The /ɚ/ in _encourage_ is also pronounced /ʌr/.

SOUND FOCUS 4: /w/

To produce the sound /w/, as in *want*, push your lips forward, rounding them tightly. Pull the back of your tongue upward toward the soft roof of the mouth Make a voiced sound as you blend the sound /w/ into the following vowel.

Underline the letters that make the sound /w/.

want	one	aware	why[3]
work	once	reward	question
well	walk	always	sway

SOUND FOCUS 5: LINKING AND HOLDING

A. Review consonant-to-vowel linking, and reduction of **and** and **h.**

before I die	looked after his dogs
What a question	puts on her shoes
When I was a child	concern and encouragement

B. First listen and then practice vowel-to-vowel linking. Use voicing to link each group of words as if it were one word.

you asked	you *oughta	the oak
go out	no one	my education

C. First listen and then practice vowel-to-consonant linking.

to do	do you	the wind
to gain	do they	we work

D. **Holding** is a form of linking. When the same consonant occurs between two words in a phrase, do not pronounce the sound twice. Pronounce it once, and hold it for a slightly longer time.

a good day	whole life	a famous scientist
a big gorilla	with three sons	you must study[4]

E. When similar consonants occur between two words in a phrase, do not release the first consonant. Release the second. Practice holding the similar consonants in these phrases.[5]

had time	Liz saw us
stooped down	both these songs

---

[3]Words spelled **wh**, such as *why, what, wheat* may be pronounced /w/ or /hw/.
[4]Note that this combination, **st-st**, becomes /st/, with the /s/ held longer.
[5]Voiceless-voiced pairs, such as /t-d/, /s-z/, /θ-ð/, /k-g/, /f-v/, /p-b/, are similar in that the position of the lips, teeth, tongue and jaw are the same.

have fun   breathe thin air

back gate   rub palms

hug Koko   clap both hands

SOUNDS IN CONTEXT: PHRASE BY PHRASE 1

Listen and put a small dot (·) over the vowel in each syllable. Then rewind the tape and practice the passage in short phrases.

"Why do you work?" | you asked me. | What a complex question! |
Do we work | to serve society | or to gain | personal satisfaction? |
Do we work to earn money | or because there's nothing better | to do? |
Perhaps no one can answer it | very well. | I'll just try to comment |
on why I work. |

When I was a child, | my mother urged me |
to further my education. | She said, "Son, | you must study hard. |
You have to become | a famous scientist | someday. | That'll be |
my reward." | My mother spent her whole life |
supporting her children. |
With three sons | and three daughters, | she had to work very hard. |
I'll never forget | her constant concern | and encouragement. |

A person lives only once. | I think | if I haven't done |
something important | before I die, | I'll certainly be sorry! |
So I want to accomplish | as much as possible. |
If I can make a small mark, | I'll feel very happy. | It'll mean |
that my life has purpose. | I've already reached |
a little success in my work | and published some articles |
on my research. | But I still want to do | much more. | As a father, |
I want to provide a good model | for my daughter. |

What's your viewpoint? |

SOUNDS IN CONTEXT: PHRASE BY PHRASE 2

Listen and underline the /w/ sounds once and the /ɚ/ sounds twice. (Note that /w/ can be written with **w, o,** or **u.** /ɚ/ can be written with **er, ir, or, ur, ar, ear,** and **our.**) Then rewind the tape and practice the passage in longer phrases.

"Why do you work?" you asked me. | What a complex question! |
Do we work to serve society | or to gain personal satisfaction? |
Do we work to earn money | or because there's nothing better to do? |
Perhaps no one can answer it very well. |
I'll just try to comment on why I work. |

When I was a child, | my mother urged me
to further my education. |

She said, "Son, you must study hard. |
You have to become a famous scientist | someday. |
That'll be my reward." | My mother spent her whole life |
supporting her children. | With three sons and three daughters, |
she had to work very hard. | I'll never forget |
her constant concern and encouragement. |

A person lives only once. | I think |
if I haven't done something important before I die, |
I'll certainly be sorry! | So I want to accomplish as much as possible. |
If I can make a small mark, | I'll feel very happy. |
It'll mean that my life has purpose. |
I've already reached a little success in my work |
and published some articles on my research. |
But I still want to do much more. | As a father, |
I want to provide a good model for my daughter. |

What's your viewpoint? |

SOUNDS IN CONTEXT: PHRASE BY PHRASE 3

Listen and underline the /ɑ/ sounds once and the /ʌ/ sounds twice. (Note that
/ɑ/ can be written with **a** and **o,** and /ʌ/ with **u, o,** and **ou.**) Then rewind the
tape and practice the passage in complete sentences.

"Why do you work?" you asked me. | What a complex question! |
Do we work to serve society or to gain personal satisfaction? |
Do we work to earn money or because there's nothing better to do? |
Perhaps no one can answer it very well. |
I'll just try to comment on why I work. |

When I was a child, my mother urged me
to further my education. | She said, "Son, you must study hard. |
You have to become a famous scientist someday. | That'll be my reward." |
My mother spent her whole life supporting her children. |
With three sons and three daughters, she had to work very hard. |
I'll never forget her constant concern and encouragement. |

A person lives only once. | I think if I haven't done
something important before I die, I'll certainly be sorry! |
So I want to accomplish as much as possible. | If I can make a small mark, |
I'll feel very happy. | It'll mean that my life has purpose. |
I've already reached a little success in my work and published some articles
on my research. | But I still want to do much more. |
As a father, I want to provide a good model for my daughter. |

What's your viewpoint? |

ON YOUR OWN

Review the **Sound Focus** exercises introduced in this lesson.
Practice **Phrase by Phrase** steps several times.
Record the passage from beginning to end without stopping.

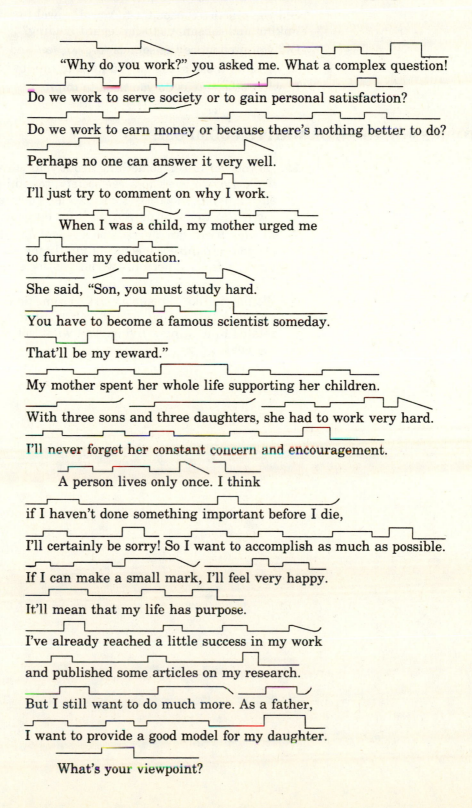

"Why do you work?" you asked me. What a complex question!

Do we work to serve society or to gain personal satisfaction?

Do we work to earn money or because there's nothing better to do?

Perhaps no one can answer it very well.

I'll just try to comment on why I work.

When I was a child, my mother urged me

to further my education.

She said, "Son, you must study hard.

You have to become a famous scientist someday.

That'll be my reward."

My mother spent her whole life supporting her children.

With three sons and three daughters, she had to work very hard.

I'll never forget her constant concern and encouragement.

A person lives only once. I think

if I haven't done something important before I die,

I'll certainly be sorry! So I want to accomplish as much as possible.

If I can make a small mark, I'll feel very happy.

It'll mean that my life has purpose.

I've already reached a little success in my work

and published some articles on my research.

But I still want to do much more. As a father,

I want to provide a good model for my daughter.

What's your viewpoint?

Listen to your recording.

Did you say the correct number of syllables?

Did you make stressed syllables longer than unstressed syllables?

Did you use appropriate rising intonation and falling intonation at the end of statements and questions?

Did you practice consonant-to-vowel, vowel-to-consonant, vowel-to-vowel linking and consonant-to-consonant holding?

Did you pronounce the sounds /ɑ/, /ʌ/, /ɝ/ and /w/ clearly?

In which of these areas do you need to improve?

In what other areas do you need to improve?

TOPICS FOR ORAL OR WRITTEN COMPOSITION

1. Do you work? Tell something about your job and the reasons why you work. Do you work to serve society, to gain personal satisfaction, to earn a living, to satisfy someone else's desires, because there's nothing better to do, or do you work for other reasons?

2. In what ways can a person be a model for others? For what reasons? Do you recognize someone—a family member, a friend, an acquaintance, a famous person—whom you look up to as a model for your life?

3. Would you like to make a mark in some field? It could be the field you are working in now, a field you want to change to, or a field not related to making a living. Tell what you would like to accomplish someday.

Chapter 10

Rafting through the Grand Canyon

VOCABULARY FOCUS

Do you or your classmates know the *italicized* words in this list? Complete each sentence with a word or phrase from the list. Change nouns and verbs to appropriate forms. Discuss your choices with a partner.

1. _____ The room was so *silent* that you could hear a pin drop.

2. _____ A *blanket* of darkness covered the fields.

3. _____ They crossed the lake on a rubber *raft*.

4. _____ Several deep *caverns* can be seen in the canyon walls.

5. _____ The dancers *whirled* around and around the dance floor.

6. _____ Let's *flip* a coin. If it's heads, I win; if it's tails, you win.

7. _____ A bottle with a message in it *floated* down the stream.

8. _____ Mrs. Finney lost her balance and *tumbled* down the stairs.

9. _____ The river turns into a waterfall where it flows over a *cliff*.

10. _____ Rafting along gentle parts of a river can be relaxing, but rafting through the white water of the *rapids* is usually more *thrilling*.

11. _____ My *adventure* traveling on a river *raft* left me with unforgettable memories.

12. _____ Our guide was an *expert* at explaining special points of interest in the scenery.

13. _____ After the rain, the sun came out and we could see a *spectacular* rainbow across the sky.

14. _____ When the airplane crashed, several passengers died, but most *survived*.

A. exciting
B. quiet
C. stayed alive
D. high steep rock
E. exciting and often dangerous trip

F. large caves
G. rode in water
H. thick covering
I. fell suddenly
J. turned around quickly

K. turn over
L. striking; magnificent
M. very skilled person
N. flat boat

BEFORE YOU LISTEN

Look at the picture and tell what you think.

Are the people rafting on a lake, a river, or an ocean?
Do they look afraid or thrilled?
Describe the scenery.
What is the man in the inset (upper right corner) looking at?

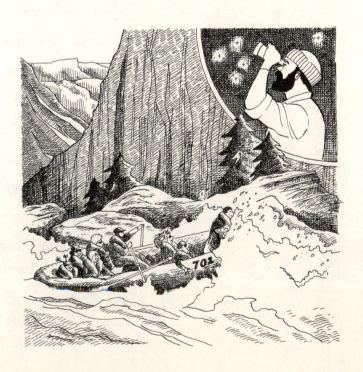

The Grand Canyon is a gorge formed by the Colorado River in northwestern Arizona (a southwestern state of the USA). In some places the canyon gets as deep as one mile. In the spring and summer, when the winter snows in the mountains have melted, the Colorado rushes through the Grand Canyon. This, along with the natural beauty of the canyon, attracted Ellen to take a rafting trip through the Grand Canyon.

LISTENING COMPREHENSION

Read these statements. Listen to the passage and choose the best answer for each statement.

1. Ellen has been floating down the Colorado River for _____.
   a. a week
   b. three or four days
   c. three or four hours
   d. four weeks

2. Tumbling through the rapids was _____.
   a. wet
   b. exciting
   c. dangerous
   d. all of the above

3. Altogether, _____ people went on the rafting trip.
   a. nine
   b. ten
   c. eleven
   d. twelve

4. She could hardly believe her eyes because _____.
   a. the scenery was so spectacular
   b. the raft trip was so dangerous
   c. the water was so cold
   d. her eyesight was so bad

5. The caverns were _____.
   a. silent
   b. white
   c. red
   d. rainbow-colored

6. They "hiked up side canyons" means _____
   a. They climbed up the cliffs
   b. They hiked up small canyons leading from the main canyon
   c. They walked up the canyons side by side
   d. They moved sideways up the canyons

7. Ellen saw _____ stars in the night sky.
   a. no
   b. a few
   c. several
   d. many

8. Ellen will _____ the Grand Canyon.
   a. not remember
   b. never forget
   c. survive in
   d. return to

LISTENING CLOZE

Listen to the passage again. Fill in the words you hear, one word for each blank. Pause the tape as necessary.

You'll never guess where I've been! I've been

(1) _____ down (2) _____

Colorado River for a week on a rubber (3) _____. I

took a trip with two (4) _____ guides and nine

other passengers. It was (5) _____ to tumble

through the (6) _____, although sometimes I wasn't

sure (7) _____ get down the river alive. A couple of

times our raft (8) _____ around and flipped

(9) _____ into the cold water. Somehow I survived

the danger and excitement! The (10) _____ in the

Grand Canyon is so spectacular that I (11) _____

hardly believe my eyes. I was amazed at the rainbow-

(12) _____ canyon walls. The deep blue sky, the red

(13) _____, and the white water made a beautiful

picture. We usually spent only three or four hours a day

(14) _____ the raft. The rest of the time we hiked

up side canyons, fished in (15) _____ streams, and

played near waterfalls. At night we (16) _____

asleep under a silent blanket of sparkling

(17) _____. Rafting through the Grand Canyon was

truly an unforgettable (18) _____.

DISCUSSION

In what ways was the scenery spectacular?
Why was Ellen sometimes unsure she'd get down the river alive?
Have you ever visited the Grand Canyon?

SOUND FOCUS 1: UNSTRESSING FUNCTION WORDS

As you have practiced in previous lessons, content words (such as nouns, main verbs, adjectives and adverbs) are generally long, strong, clear and high.

Function words are usually *unstressed* when spoken in phrases. This means that they are *short, weak, unclear,* and *low*.

Function words include articles, prepositions, conjunctions, auxiliary verbs and personal pronouns. They also include possessive adjectives, relative pronouns and adverbs, and simple forms of the verb *be*.

First listen to the following phrases. Notice how the function words, which are crossed out, are shorter, weaker, less clear, and lower than the content words. Then go back and practice.

~~I was~~ too busy dancing ~~and~~ singing.

How good ~~are you at~~ using chopsticks?

growing ~~on the~~ rim ~~of the~~ river

~~If I can~~ make ~~a~~ small mark

~~his~~ heart ~~would be~~ shaken ~~out of his~~ body

~~You'll~~ never guess ~~where I've~~ been

~~A~~ couple ~~of~~ times ~~our~~ raft whirled around

~~as if he were a~~ baby gorilla

SOUND FOCUS 2: RHYTHM

The alternation of stressed and unstressed syllables creates a **rhythm** that sounds distinctly English. In the example below, the length of the line above each syllable indicates how long it is pronounced in relation to the others.

‾ . ——— —— . —— . . ———
I was too busy dancing and singing.

Go back to the sentences in **Sound Focus 1.** Repeat the phrases. At the same time, mark the beat by clapping your hands together at each syllable.

SOUND FOCUS 3: THOUGHT PHRASES

English speakers group words together in phrases that make sense as **thought groups.** Stress (making a syllable strong), intonation (changing the pitch) and pausing (stopping briefly) are used to indicate the end of a phrase.

A. First, listen to, then practice the following patterns for American telephone numbers.

999-9999 →   nine nine níne | nine níne | nine níne |

444-4444 →   four four fóur | four fóur | four fóur |

If you have a telephone number, a student number, a social security number, a credit card number, etc., practice saying it to a partner.

B. Look at the phrasing in the following sentences. Which phrasing divides the words into appropriate thought groups?

1. a. She gave me | a red dress.

   b. She gave | me a red | dress.

2. a. I'll see | you on Saturday.

   b. I'll see you | on Saturday.

3. a. Do you have to pay | at the door?

   b. Do you have | to pay at | the door?

4. a. Mom and Dad are | going away.

   b. Mom and Dad | are going away.

Some common logical patterns of phrasing are: compound subject, verb phrase, subject + verb, subject + verb + object, modifiers + noun, prepositional phrase.

C. Working with a partner, divide the following sentences into thought group phrases.

You'll never guess where I've been! I've been floating down the Colorado River for a week on a rubber raft. I took a trip with two expert guides and nine other passengers.

Go back to the **Listening Cloze** of this lesson and continue to group the words into thought phrases.

SOUND FOCUS 4: /r/

To produce the sound /r/, as in _raft,_ raise your tongue and curl it toward the hard roof of your mouth.[1] Let the sides of your tongue touch the upper side teeth. Do not let the tip of your tongue touch anything (the roof of your mouth, your teeth, etc.). Round your lips slightly. Make a voiced sound.

A. In the following words, pronounce the vowel clearly before moving the tongue backward into position for the sound /r/.

Underline the letters that make the /r/ sound.

are	oar	ears	forest
car	more	corn	carry
air	poor	tired	hurry
fare	hour	heart	starry

B. You will recall that the tongue is also curled to pronounce the sound /ɚ/, as in _earn_. Remember that /ɚ/ forms a syllable while /r/ does not. Listen to these words and check (√) the sound you hear.

---

[1]See Footnote #1 in Lesson 9, _Why I Work_

	/ɚ/	vowel + /r/		/ɚ/	vowel + /r/
word	✓	____	start	____	____
four	____	____	purple	____	____
birth	____	____	cavern	____	____
farm	____	____	water	____	____

C. In the following words, curl the tongue in position before letting it blend into the following vowel sound. Take care not to let the tip of your tongue touch anything.

raft	rest	around	grand
rapids	rainbow	arrive	trip
rock	river	parade	through
red	rubber	erase	streams

SOUND FOCUS 5: /l/

To produce the sound /l/, as in *lake,* place the tip of your tongue on the upper gum ridge and leave the middle of your tongue in a low to mid position. Do not let the sides of your tongue touch anything. Keep your lips relaxed; do not round them. Let a voiced breath come over the relaxed sides of the tongue.

A. In the following words, pronounce the vowel clearly before moving the tip of your tongue onto the gum ridge for the sound /l/. Leave the middle of your tongue in a low to mid position.

Underline the letters that make the /l/ sound.

all	fell	cold	little
fall	he'll	child	it'll
small	I'll	although	couple
hole	you'll	beautiful	tumble

B. In the following words, place the tip of your tongue on the gum ridge for the sound /l/ before letting it blend into the following vowel sound.

leave	lawn	believe	blanket
living	lower	alive	floating
let	love	colored	asleep
laugh	life	only	played

SOUNDS IN CONTEXT: PHRASE BY PHRASE 1

Listen and cross out the unstressed function words. Then rewind the tape and practice the passage in short phrases. While you speak, clap out the rhythm.

~~You'll~~ never guess | ~~where I've~~ been! | ~~I've been~~ floating |
down the Colorado River | for a week | on a rubber raft. | I took a trip |
with two expert guides | and nine other passengers. | It was thrilling |
to tumble through the rapids, | although sometimes | I wasn't sure |
I'd get down the river | alive. | A couple of times |
our raft whirled around | and flipped over | into the cold water. |
Somehow I survived | the danger and excitement! | The scenery |
in the Grand Canyon | is so spectacular | that I could hardly |
believe my eyes. | I was amazed | at the rainbow-colored |
canyon walls. | The deep blue sky, | the red caverns, |
and the white water | made a beautiful picture. | We usually spent |
only three or four hours a day | on the raft. | The rest of the time |
we hiked up side canyons, | fished in small streams, |
and played near waterfalls. | At night | we fell asleep |
under a silent blanket | of sparkling stars. |
Rafting through the Grand Canyon | was truly | an unforgettable |
adventure. |

SOUNDS IN CONTEXT: PHRASE BY PHRASE 2

Listen and underline the /ɚ/ sounds once and the *vowel* + /r/ sounds twice. (Note that /ɚ/ can be written with **er, ir, or, ar** or **ur.**) Rewind the tape and practice the passage in longer phrases.

You'll nev<u>er</u> guess wh<u><u>ere</u></u> I've been! |
I've been floating down the Colorado River |
for a week on a rubber raft. | I took a trip with two expert guides |
and nine other passengers. |
It was thrilling to tumble through the rapids, |
although sometimes I wasn't sure | I'd get down the river alive. |
A couple of times | our raft whirled around and flipped over |
into the cold water. | Somehow I survived the danger and excitement! |
The scenery in the Grand Canyon | is so spectacular |
that I could hardly believe my eyes. | I was amazed |
at the rainbow-colored canyon walls. |
The deep blue sky, the red caverns, and the white water |
made a beautiful picture. |
We usually spent only three or four hours a day | on the raft. |
The rest of the time we hiked up side canyons, |
fished in small streams, and played near waterfalls. |

At night we fell asleep | under a silent blanket of sparkling stars. |
Rafting through the Grand Canyon |
was truly an unforgettable adventure. |

SOUNDS IN CONTEXT: PHRASE BY PHRASE 3

Listen and underline the /l/ sounds. (Note that some **l** letters are silent.)
Rewind the tape and practice the passage in complete sentences.

You'll never guess where I've been! | I've been floating down
the Colorado River for a week on a rubber raft. |
I took a trip with two expert guides and nine other passengers. |
It was thrilling to tumble through the rapids, although sometimes
I wasn't sure I'd get down the river alive. | A couple of times
our raft whirled around and flipped over into the cold water. |
Somehow I survived the danger and excitement! |
The scenery in the Grand Canyon is so spectacular that I could hardly
believe my eyes. | I was amazed at the rainbow-colored canyon walls. |
The deep blue sky, the red caverns, and the white water
made a beautiful picture. | We usually spent only three or four hours a day
on the raft. | The rest of the time we hiked up side canyons,
fished in small streams, and played near waterfalls. |
At night we fell asleep under a silent blanket of sparkling stars. |
Rafting through the Grand Canyon
was truly an unforgettable adventure. |

ON YOUR OWN

Review the **Sound Focus** exercises introduced in this lesson.
Practice **Phrase by Phrase** steps several times.
Record the passage on the next page from beginning to end without
stopping.

You'll <u>never</u> <u>guess</u> <u>where</u> I've <u>been</u>! I've been <u>floating</u>

down the Colo<u>ra</u>do <u>River</u> for a <u>week</u> on a <u>rubber</u> <u>raft</u>.

I <u>took</u> a <u>trip</u> with <u>two</u> <u>expert</u> <u>guides</u> and <u>nine</u> <u>other</u> pa<u>ss</u>engers.

It was <u>thrilling</u> to <u>tumble</u> through the <u>rapids</u>,

although <u>sometimes</u> I wasn't <u>sure</u> I'd <u>get</u> down the <u>river</u> a<u>live</u>.

A <u>couple</u> of <u>times</u> our <u>raft</u> <u>whirled</u> a<u>round</u>

and <u>flipped</u> <u>o</u>ver into the <u>cold</u> <u>water</u>.

<u>Somehow</u> I sur<u>vived</u> the <u>danger</u> and ex<u>cite</u>ment!

The <u>scenery</u> in the <u>Grand</u> <u>Canyon</u> is <u>so</u> spec<u>ta</u>cular

that I could <u>hardly</u> be<u>lieve</u> my <u>eyes</u>.

I was a<u>mazed</u> at the <u>rainbow-colored</u> <u>canyon</u> <u>walls</u>. The <u>deep</u> <u>blue</u> <u>sky</u>,

the <u>red</u> <u>caverns</u>, and the <u>white</u> <u>water</u> <u>made</u> a <u>beautiful</u> <u>picture</u>.

We <u>usually</u> <u>spent</u> <u>only</u> <u>three</u> or <u>four</u> <u>hours</u> a <u>day</u> on the <u>raft</u>.

The <u>rest</u> of the <u>time</u> we <u>hiked</u> up <u>side</u> <u>canyons</u>, <u>fished</u> in <u>small</u> <u>streams</u>,

and <u>played</u> near <u>waterfalls</u>.

At <u>night</u> we <u>fell</u> a<u>sleep</u> under a <u>silent</u> <u>blanket</u> of <u>sparkling</u> <u>stars</u>.

<u>Raft</u>ing through the <u>Grand</u> <u>Canyon</u>

was <u>truly</u> an unfor<u>get</u>table ad<u>ven</u>ture.

Listen to your recording.

Did you say words together in thought phrases?
Did you make the content words longer and clearer than the function words?
Did you make the function words shorter, weaker, and less clear than the content words?
Did you pronounce the sounds /l/ and /r/ clearly?
Did you make a difference between /ɚ/ and *vowel* + /r/?
Did you make a distinction between clear and reduced vowels?
In which of these areas do you need to improve?
In what other areas do you need to improve?

TOPICS FOR ORAL OR WRITTEN COMPOSITION

1. Have you had an exciting or thrilling adventure? Tell where you went, what you saw, how you felt, and how it was different from other experiences you have had.
2. Have you ever ridden a boat down a river or across a sea? Describe your trip. Was it similar to or different from Ellen's rafting trip down the Colorado River?
3. Find out more about Grand Canyon National Park. Tell why this place attracts people to visit it.

Chapter 11

The Accident

VOCABULARY FOCUS

Do you or your classmates know the words in this list? Complete each sentence with a word or phrase from the list. Change nouns and verbs to appropriate forms. Discuss your choices with a partner.

accident	bruised	glare	sheepishly
ambulance	daydream	hop	sneak up
avoid	end up	horn	supermarket
bicyclist	excuse	howl	tune
blare			

1. A driver drives a car; a _____ rides a bicycle.

2. Two cars crashed into each other. Fortunately, nobody was hurt in the _____.

3. To _____ catching a cold, stay healthy and warm.

4. A driver pushes the _____ in a car to make a loud warning noise.

5. Who is making that long, loud cry? It sounds like the _____ of a wild animal.

6. A _____ sells all kinds of food and goods.

7. An _____ took the injured people to the hospital.

8. Did he stand up slowly or did he _____ up from his seat?

9. My neighbors play loud, sharp, unpleasant music. I can't stand it when the music _____ from their window.

10. He _____ at me with angry eyes.

11. Is your leg _____? It's all black and blue.

12. "I'm ashamed of my foolish mistake," she said _____.

13. I started out taking Math 2, but because I failed all of my tests, I _____ going back to Math 1.

14. Sometimes when I am awake, I imagine that I am somewhere else: I _____.

15. The thief _____ behind me on the bus and picked my pocket.

16. You said you didn't do your homework because you were absent yesterday. Is that a good _____?

17. I can remember the words to that song, but I can't remember the _____.

BEFORE YOU LISTEN

Look at the picture and tell what you think.

Where is the woman?
Where is the man?
What happened?

Cars are both common and important in America. People drive to work, to school, to the store, to the bank, to shows, on trips, and simply for pleasure. There are even many popular songs about driving. In contrast, bicycles are much less common. Bicycles must follow the same traffic rules as cars, but because of the difference in size and speed, these two kinds of vehicles sometimes run into trouble on the road.

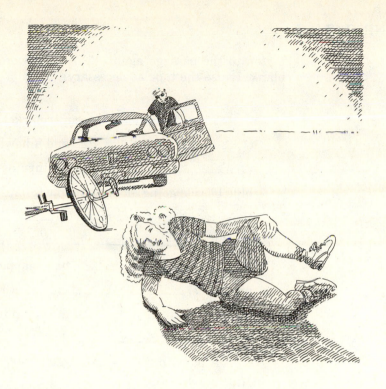

LISTENING COMPREHENSION

Read these statements. Listen to the passage and choose the best answer for each statement.

1. The collision happened at the entrance to a parking lot.
   a. True   b. False   c. We can't tell

2. The car and the bicycle were going in opposite directions.
   a. True   b. False   c. We can't tell

3. The driver couldn't believe he had struck the bicyclist.
   a. True   b. False   c. We can't tell

4. The bicyclist glared at the driver.
   a. True   b. False   c. We can't tell

5. The driver got out of his car slowly.
   a. True   b. False   c. We can't tell

6. The police officer turned down the driver's radio.
   a. True   b. False   c. We can't tell

7. The driver likes music.
   a. True   b. False   c. We can't tell

8. The bicyclist likes music.
   a. True   b. False   c. We can't tell

9. The police officer took the bicyclist to the hospital.
   a. True   b. False   c. We can't tell

LISTENING CLOZE

Listen to the passage again. Fill in the words you hear, one word for each blank. Pause the tape as necessary.

Yesterday outside the supermarket, I heard the sounds of a

(1) _____ and a howl. A

(2) _____ car turning right into the parking lot hit a

blue bicycle going along the same (3) _____. When

the driver hopped out, music (4) _____ from his car.

He (5) _____ his head and said, "This

(6) _____ have happened!" The woman lying on the

ground (7) _____ at him. "You must have

(8) _____ daydreaming. It shouldn't have

(9) _____, but it did!"

A police officer came to take a report. "Sir,"

(10) _____ said to the driver,

"(11) _____ you please turn down your radio? I can

(12) _____ hear." He turned it down, yelling, "She

shouldn't have (13) _____ up behind me!"

"What a fool!" replied the bicyclist. "If

(14) _____ been paying attention, maybe you would

(15) _____ seen me! And I wouldn't have ended up

hurt and (16) _____." At that point, the red-faced

driver stooped down and (17) _____ her to her feet.

"They were playing my favorite tune," he said sheepishly.

"Horrible (18) _____!" she answered. As an

(19) _____ took the woman to the hospital, I thought

about how a good driver would have (20) _____ this

accident.

DISCUSSION

How did this accident happen?
Was it anybody's fault?
Why was the driver red-faced?
Could the collision have been avoided?

SOUND FOCUS 1: /u^w/

To produce the sound /u^w/, as in *shoe,* round your lips tightly and raise the back of your tongue toward the soft roof of the mouth. As you make a voiced sound, pull **your** tongue upward and backwards and push your lips forward, gliding into a /w/ sound: /u^w/.

Underline the letters that make the sound /u^w/.

sh<u>oe</u>	fool	students[1]
b<u>oo</u>m	youth	cooler
stoop	new	supermarket
blue	tune	consumer

SOUND FOCUS 2: /ʊ/

To produce the sound /ʊ/, as in *p<u>u</u>t,* round your lips slightly (but less than for /u^w/) and raise the back of your tongue high (but slightly lower and more relaxed than for /u^w/). Do not move your tongue or lips. Make a voiced sound.

Underline the letters that make the sound /ʊ/.

p<u>u</u>t	shook	woman
should	foot	couldn't
good	stood	wouldn't
push	pull	sugar

SOUND FOCUS 3: /y/

To produce the sound /y/, as in *yes,* raise the middle of your tongue to a high position, as for the sound /i/. Make the muscles of your cheeks and tongue tense. As you make a voiced sound, let your tongue glide into the following vowel sound. Do not let your tongue touch the roof of your mouth.

Underline the letters that make the sound /y/.[2]

<u>y</u>es	canyon	excuse
year	onion	usually
yard	few	regular
union	beautiful	population

---

[1]The /u^w/ in *new, tune, students, supermarket,* and *consumer* may also be pronounced /yu^u/.

[2]Note that the sound /y/ often precedes /u^w/, /ʊ/, and /ə/ to form /yu^w/, /yʊ/, and /yə/.

SOUND FOCUS 4: REDUCTION: CONDITIONALS

A. Practice contracting and reducing the auxiliary verb *had* to *'d* or **'id*.

Mom had never seen her.
→   *Mommid never *seener.

Bob had driven there once.
→   *Bobbid driven there once.

If you had been paying attention . . .
→   If you'd been paying attention

If it had happened at night . . .
→   If it'd happened at night   (it'd → *itid)

If the woman had died . . .
→   If the *womanid died

B. When the modals *should, could, would, must, may,* and *might* are followed by *have* + past participle, the auxiliary *have* is usually contracted so that it sounds like *of (/əv/). It is also commonly reduced even further before a consonant so that it sounds like *a (/ə/). Listen first to the careful and formal pronunciation of the following sentences, and then to the relaxed, informal reductions.

They might have avoided the collision.
→   They *might-of avoided the collision.

She could have eaten more.
→   She *could-of eaten more.

You should have been paying attention.
→   You *should-of been paying attention.
⟶   You *shoulda been paying attention.

I would have gone, but I didn't have time.
→   I *would-of gone, but I didn't have time.
⟶   I *woulda gone, but I didn't have time.

You must have been daydreaming.
→   You *must-of been daydreaming.
⟶   You *musta been daydreaming.

C. The negative *not have* is often reduced to *'int-of or *ina in relaxed, informal speech.

I wouldn't have ended up like this.
→   I *wouldint-of ended up like this.

He mustn't have understood.
→   He *mussint-of understood.

It couldn't have happened.
→   It *couldint-of happened.
⟶   It *couldina happened.

They shouldn't have collided.
→   They *shouldint-of collided.
⟶   They *shouldina collided.

SOUND FOCUS 5: STRESS AND TIMING

A. English is a **stress-timed** language. Stresses tend to recur at regular intervals of time. This tendency combines with word stress variation to make English rhythm distinct from other languages.[3] In the following examples, notice how the unstressed syllables are shortened to fit in between stressed syllables.

1.

a níce   dáy
a prétty   dáy
a beáutiful dáy
a spectácular dáy

2.

a máth   téacher
an Énglish téacher
a chémistry téacher
a philósophy téacher

3.

I wón't   taĺk.
I dídn't   taĺk.
I cóuldn't have   taĺked.
I shóuldn't have been   taĺking.

4.

He ásked   a quéstion.
He ánswered a quéstion.
He repéated a quéstion.
He intérpreted a quéstion.

B. Practice saying these phrases to a partner, keeping the same stress and timing in each set.

1.

a néw blúe hát
a new blue sweater
a new orange sweater
a pretty orange sweater

2.

I cán't sée her
I couldn't see her
I couldn't have seen her
I couldn't have talked to her

---

[3]Compared with English and other Germanic languages, French, for example, is a **syllable-timed** language. In French, syllables, rather than only stressed syllables, tend to recur at regular intervals.

SOUNDS IN CONTEXT: PHRASE BY PHRASE 1

Listen and underline the /uʷ/ sounds once and the /ʊ/ sounds twice. (Note that /uʷ/ sounds can be spelled **u, oo, o, ui, ew, eu, ue,** and **ou.** /ʊ/ can be spelled **u, oo,** and **ou.**) Then rewind the tape and practice the passage in short phrases.

Yesterday | outside the supermarket, | I heard the sounds |
of a horn and a howl. | A yellow car turning right | into the parking lot |
hit a blue bicycle | going along the same avenue. |
When the driver hopped out, | music blared from his car. |
He shook his head and said, | "This couldn't have happened!" |
The woman lying on the ground | glared at him. |
"You must have been daydreaming. | It shouldn't have happened, |
but it did!" |

A police officer | came to take a report. | "Sir," |
she said to the driver, | "would you please | turn down your radio? |
I can hardly hear." | He turned it down, | yelling, |
"She shouldn't have sneaked up | behind me!" |

"What a fool!" | replied the bicyclist. |
"If you'd been paying attention, | maybe | you would have seen me! |
And I wouldn't have ended up | hurt and bruised." |

At that point, | the red-faced driver stooped down |
and pulled her to her feet. | "They were playing my favorite tune," |
he said sheepishly. |

"Horrible excuse!" | she answered. |
As an ambulance took the woman | to the hospital, |
I thought about how a good driver | would have avoided |
this accident. |

SOUNDS IN CONTEXT: PHRASE BY PHRASE 2

Listen and underline the /h/ sounds. Draw a slash (/) through the reduced **h** letters (the ones that have disappeared). Draw a circle around the /y/ sounds. Note that not all **y** letters are pronounced /y/, and that some /y/ sounds are "hidden" in other letters. Then rewind the tape and practice the passage in longer phrases.

Ⓨesterday outside the supermarket, |

I heard the sounds of a horn and a howl. |

A yellow car turning right into the parking lot |

hit a blue bicycle going along the same avenue. |

When the driver hopped out, | music blared from his car. |

He shook his head and said, | "This couldn't have happened!" |

The woman lying on the ground glared at him. |

"You must have been daydreaming. | It shouldn't have happened, | but it did!" |

A police officer came to take a report. |

"Sir," she said to the driver, | "would you please turn down your radio? | I can hardly hear." |

He turned it down, yelling, | "She shouldn't have sneaked up behind me.!" |

"What a fool!" | replied the bicyclist. |

"If you'd been paying attention, | maybe you would have seen me! | And I wouldn't have ended up hurt and bruised." |

At that point, | the red-faced driver stooped down and pulled her to her feet. |

"They were playing my favorite tune," | he said sheepishly. |

"Horrible excuse!" she answered. |

As an ambulance took the woman to the hospital, | I thought about how a good driver | would have avoided this accident. |

SOUNDS IN CONTEXT: PHRASE BY PHRASE 3

Mark the places where linking occurs. Then rewind the tape and practice the passage in complete sentences.

Yesterday outside the supermarket,
I heard the sounds of a horn and a howl. |
A yellow car turning right into the parking lot
hit a blue bicycle going along the same avenue. |
When the driver hopped out, music blared from his car. |
He shook his head and said, "This couldn't have happened!" |
The woman lying on the ground glared at him. |
"You must have been daydreaming. | It shouldn't have happened,
but it did!" |
A police officer came to take a report. | "Sir,"
she said to the driver, "would you please turn down your radio? |
I can hardly hear." | He turned it down, yelling,
"She shouldn't have sneaked up behind me!" |
"What a fool!" replied the bicyclist. |
"If you'd been paying attention, maybe you would have seen me! |
And I wouldn't have ended up hurt and bruised." | At that point,
the red-faced driver stooped down and pulled her to her feet. |
"They were playing my favorite tune," he said sheepishly. |
"Horrible excuse!" she answered. |
As an ambulance took the woman to the hospital,
I thought about how a good driver would have avoided this accident. |

ON YOUR OWN

Review the **Sound Focus** exercises introduced in this lesson.
Practice **Phrase by Phrase** steps several times.
Record the passage from beginning to end without stopping.

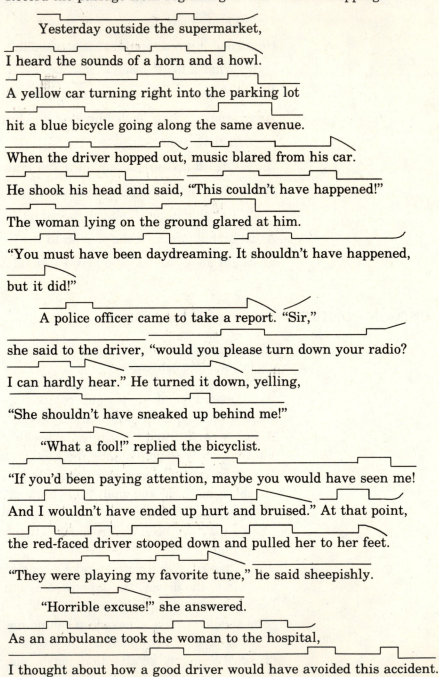

Yesterday outside the supermarket,

I heard the sounds of a horn and a howl.

A yellow car turning right into the parking lot

hit a blue bicycle going along the same avenue.

When the driver hopped out, music blared from his car.

He shook his head and said, "This couldn't have happened!"

The woman lying on the ground glared at him.

"You must have been daydreaming. It shouldn't have happened,

but it did!"

A police officer came to take a report. "Sir,"

she said to the driver, "would you please turn down your radio?

I can hardly hear." He turned it down, yelling,

"She shouldn't have sneaked up behind me!"

"What a fool!" replied the bicyclist.

"If you'd been paying attention, maybe you would have seen me!

And I wouldn't have ended up hurt and bruised." At that point,

the red-faced driver stooped down and pulled her to her feet.

"They were playing my favorite tune," he said sheepishly.

"Horrible excuse!" she answered.

As an ambulance took the woman to the hospital,

I thought about how a good driver would have avoided this accident.

Listen to your recording.

Did you group words together in thought phrases?

Did you make the content words longer and higher than the function words?

Did you shorten and weaken the unstressed syllables to fit between the stressed syllables?

Did you follow the stress patterns indicated above?

Did you reduce the auxiliaries in conditional phrases?

Did you pronounce the sounds /y/, /uᵂ/ and /ʊ/ clearly?

Did you make a distinction between the sounds /uᵂ/ and /ʊ/, /uᵂ/ and /yuᵂ/?

TOPICS FOR ORAL OR WRITTEN COMPOSITION

1. Have you ever been in a traffic accident? Describe what happened. Could it have been avoided? Describe what should have happened.

2. Have you ever done anything that you wish you hadn't done? Tell what happened and how the situation might have been different if you had acted or thought differently.

3. Discuss one aspect of automobile safety. How can a person be a safe driver? What safety regulation(s) do you consider especially important and why?

Chapter 12

Volcanoes in the Ring of Fire

VOCABULARY FOCUS

Do you or your classmates know the words in this list? Write each word in the list next to its definition. Discuss your choices with a partner.

ash	decade	geology	severe
active	destruction	measure	volcano
avalanche	erupt	mountain range	wheat
crops	explode	mud	zone
damage	fortunately		

1. _____ a period of ten years

2. _____ luckily, successfully

3. _____ soft, sticky, wet earth

4. _____ very harmful

5. _____ ruination

6. _____ to blow up or burst

7. _____ to pour out fire with force or violence

8. _____ to find the size, length, amount, degree, etc. of something

9. _____ plants such as grain, fruit, or vegetables grown or produced by a farmer

10. _____ a grain which is often made into powder and then made into bread, noodles, and such.

11. _____ a connected line of mountains or hills

12. _____ the scientific study of the earth: its origin, history and structure

13. _____ a mountain with a large opening at the top (crater), through which melting rock (lava), steam, and gases escape with strong force from inside the earth

14. _____ the soft gray powder that remains after something has been burned

15. _____ a large mass of snow and ice crashing down the side of a mountain

16. _____ alive, functioning, able to produce the expected results

17. _____ harm, loss

18. _____ an area marked off from others by particular qualities

BEFORE YOU LISTEN

Look at the picture and tell what you think.

What ocean is shown on the map?
What continents are shown?
What volcano is shown?

Volcanoes occur in many parts of the world. Most of them occur in the region shown on the map. Because they erupt with huge force, and often quite suddenly, volcanoes can be very destructive. If geologists can predict when a volcano will erupt, they can warn people ahead of time so the damage will be lessened. Many things were damaged when Mount St. Helens erupted, but there were also a few benefits.

LISTENING COMPREHENSION

Read these statements. Listen to the passage and choose the best answer for each statement.

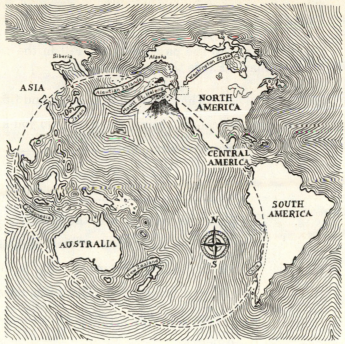

1. There are about _____ active volcanoes around the world.
   a. 815
   b. 518
   c. 850
   d. 1980

2. The "Ring of Fire" is a _____ zone.
   a. political
   b. geological
   c. historical
   d. cultural

3. _____ of the world's active volcanoes are found within the "Ring of Fire."
   a. 20%
   b. 25%
   c. 67%
   d. 75%

4. Mount St. Helens is located in _____.
   a. Alaska
   b. Washington
   c. Indonesia
   d. South America

5. Although geologists had studied the Cascade Mountain Range for several decades, they didn't realize _____.
   a. Mount St. Helens was located there
   b. Mount St. Helens was a volcano
   c. Mount St. Helens was going to erupt soon
   d. Mount St. Helens was going to erupt with such force

6. When Mount St. Helens blew up, _____.
   a. avalanches occurred
   b. plants died
   c. buildings were damaged
   d. all of the above

7. The volcanic ash was good for _____
   a. wheat and apples
   b. animals and people
   c. plants and animals
   d. roads and bridges

LISTENING CLOZE

Listen to the passage again. Fill in the words you hear, one word for each blank. Pause the tape as necessary.

There are eight hundred and fifty (1) _____ volcanoes around the world. Do you know where these mountains of fire are found? Three (2) _____ of them are found within a (3) _____ called the "Ring of Fire." One (4) _____ of the zone (5) _____ along the west coast of the Americas from Chile to Alaska. The other edge runs along the east coast of (6) _____ from Siberia to New Zealand. Twenty percent (7) _____ these volcanoes are located in Indonesia. Other big groupings are in Japan, the Aleutian (8) _____, and Central America.

In May 1980, Mount Saint Helens (9) _____ its top in Washington State. The huge (10) _____ came as a great surprise to (11) _____. They'd measured the Cascade Mountain Range for several (12) _____. But they (13) _____ expected so much destruction. The (14) _____ of Mount St. Helens sent hot volcanic (15) _____ and gases into the air. It caused (16) _____ mud slides and avalanches. It killed trees, crops, animals, and people. It (17) _____ roads, buildings, and bridges. Fortunately, not everything was (18) _____: wheat and apples grew very well in the volcanic ash.

DISCUSSION

What part of the world does the Ring of Fire include?
Which area within this zone has the most volcanoes?
Have you seen a volcanic eruption?

SOUND FOCUS 1: /ʃ/

To produce the sound /ʃ/, as in _show_, raise the sides of your tongue so that they touch the gum ridge on the sides of your teeth. Put your teeth nearly together and separate your lips. Let your voiceless breath flow out continuously through the passage between your teeth.

Listen and underline the letters that make the /ʃ/ sound.

she	ash	wishing	ocean
shade	dish	special	eruption
show	crash	machine	destruction
shoe	wash	Washington	Aleutian

SOUND FOCUS 2: /ʒ/

To produce the sound /ʒ/, as in *measure,* place your tongue, teeth and lips in the same position as for /ʃ/, described above. Let out a continuous voiced sound.

Listen and underline the letters that make the /ʒ/ sound.

measure	garage	Asia	decision
usual	rouge	Indonesia	explosion
casual	leisure	Malaysia	invasion

SOUND FOCUS 3: /tʃ/

The sound /tʃ/, as in *chair,* is a combination of the sounds /t/ and /ʃ/. To produce this sound, raise the sides of your tongue so that they touch the gum ridge on the sides of your teeth, as for the sound /ʃ/. Press the tip of your tongue against the upper gum ridge behind the front teeth, as for the sound /t/. Force air outward and let your voiceless breath explode as you quickly move the tip of your tongue away from the gum ridge.

Listen and underline the letters that make the /tʃ/ sound.

cheese	each	picture	stretches
chair	catch	natural	avalanches
Chile	march	inches	fortunately
China	watch	kitchen	actually

SOUND FOCUS 4: /dʒ/

The sound /dʒ/, as in *jail,* is a combination of the sounds /d/ and /ʒ/. To produce this sound, place your tongue, teeth and lips in the same position as for /tʒ/, /tʃ/, described above. This time, force a voiced sound to explode from your mouth as you release the tip of your tongue from its position against the gum ridge. Listen and underline the letters that make the /dʒ/ sound.

jail	edge	region	judge
joke	huge	subject	George
juice	range	bridges	geology
giant	damage	manager	geologist

SOUND FOCUS 5: SOUND AND STRESS SHIFTS

A. Consonant and vowel sounds often change systematically within word families, depending on whether the word is a noun, verb, adjective or adverb.

Listen and underline the part of the word where there is a change in consonant or vowel sound.

explode	explosion	explosive	explosively
include	inclusion	inclusive	inclusivly
receive	reception	receptive	receptively

B. Word stress can also change from one syllable to another. Listen and note the stress changes in the following patterns.

geology	geologist	geological	geologically
psychology	psychologist	psychological	psychologically
economy	economist	economical	economically
phonology	phonologist	phonological	phonologically
anatomy	anatomist	anatomical	anatomically
astronomy	astronomer	astronomical	astronomically
geography	geographer	geographical	geographically

C. Take turns saying the following words to a partner, marking the syllables and word stress. Use the stress shift patterns above as a guide.

conclude, conclusive, conclusively

perception, perceptively, perceive

biology, biologist, biological

biographical, biographer, biographically

technological, technology, technologically

SOUNDS IN CONTEXT: PHRASE BY PHRASE 1

Listen and underline the /ʃ/ sounds once and the /ʒ/ sounds twice. (Note that /ʃ/ sounds can be written with **sh, ch, ci, ce,** and **ti,** and /ʒ/ sounds with **su, ge,** and **si.**) Then rewind the tape and practice the passage in short phrases.

There are eight hundred and fifty | active volcanoes |
around the world. | Do you know | where these mountains of fire |
are found? | Three quarters of them | are found within a zone |
called the "Ring of Fire." | One edge of the zone |
stretches along the west coast | of the Americas |
from Chile to Alaska. | The other edge | runs along the east coast |
of Asia | from Siberia to New Zealand. | Twenty percent |
of these volcanoes | are located in Indonesia. | Other big groupings |
are in Japan, | the Aleutian Islands, | and Central America. |
In May 1980, | Mount Saint Helens | blew its top |
in Washington State. | The huge explosion | came as a great surprise |
to geologists. | They'd measured | the Cascade Mountain Range |
for several decades. | But they hadn't expected | so much destruction. |
The eruption of Mount St. Helens | sent hot volcanic ash and gases |
into the air. | It caused severe mud slides | and avalanches. |
It killed trees, crops, | animals, and people. |
It damaged roads, buildings, | and bridges. | Fortunately, |
not everything was lost: | wheat and apples grew very well |
in the volcanic ash.

SOUNDS IN CONTEXT: PHRASE BY PHRASE 2

Listen and underline the /tʃ/ sounds once and the /dʒ/ sounds twice. (Note that /tʃ/ sounds can be written with **ch, tch,** and **tu,** and /dʒ/ with **j, g, ge, dge,** and **gi.**) Then rewind the tape and practice the passage in longer phrases.

There are eight hundred and fifty active volcanoes |
around the world. | Do you know |
where these mountains of fire are found? |
Three quarters of them are found |
within a zone called the "Ring of Fire." | One edge of the zone |
stretches along the west coast of the Americas | from Chile to Alaska. |
The other edge | runs along the east coast of Asia |
from Siberia to New Zealand. | Twenty percent of these volcanoes |
are located in Indonesia. | Other big groupings are in Japan, |
the Aleutian Islands, | and Central America. |
In May 1980, | Mount Saint Helens blew its top |
in Washington State. | The huge explosion |
came as a great surprise to geologists. |
They'd measured the Cascade Mountain Range | for several decades. |

But they hadn't expected | so much destruction. |
The eruption of Mount St. Helens |
sent hot volcanic ash and gases into the air. |
It caused severe mud slides and avalanches. |
It killed trees, crops, animals, and people. |
It damaged roads, buildings, and bridges. |
Fortunately, not everything was lost: |
wheat and apples grew very well in the volcanic ash.

SOUNDS IN CONTEXT: PHRASE BY PHRASE 3

Listen and underline the content words and mark the phrase stress. Then rewind the tape and practice the passage in complete sentences.

There are eight hundred and fifty active volcanoes
around the world. |
Do you know where these mountains of fire are found?
| Three quarters of them are found
within a zone called the "Ring of Fire." |
One edge of the zone stretches along the west coast of the Americas
from Chile to Alaska. | The other edge runs along the east coast of Asia
from Siberia to New Zealand. | Twenty percent of these volcanoes
are located in Indonesia. | Other big groupings are in Japan,
the Aleutian Islands, and Central America. |

In May 1980, Mount Saint Helens blew its top
in Washington State. | The huge explosion came as a great surprise
to geologists. | They'd measured the Cascade Mountain Range for
several decades. | But they hadn't expected so much destruction. |
The eruption of Mount St. Helens sent hot volcanic ash and gases
into the air. | It caused severe mud slides and avalanches. |
It killed trees, crops, animals, and people. | It damaged roads,
buildings, and bridges. | Fortunately, not everything was lost: |
wheat and apples grew very well in the volcanic ash. |

ON YOUR OWN

Review the **Sound Focus** exercises introduced in this lesson.
Practice **Phrase by Phrase** steps several times.
Record the passage from beginning to end without stopping.

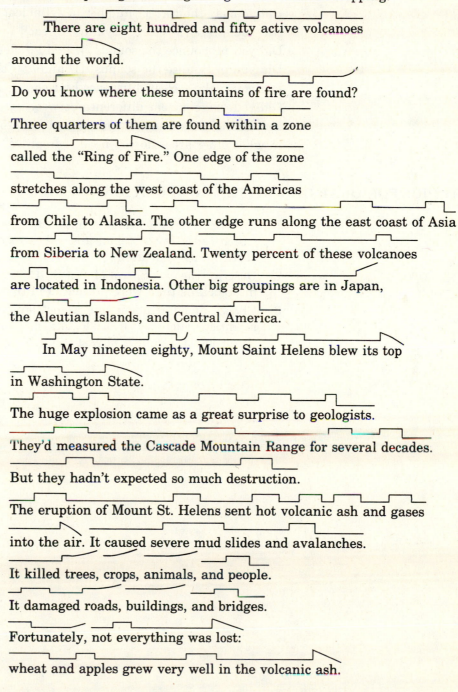

There are eight hundred and fifty active volcanoes

around the world.

Do you know where these mountains of fire are found?

Three quarters of them are found within a zone

called the "Ring of Fire." One edge of the zone

stretches along the west coast of the Americas

from Chile to Alaska. The other edge runs along the east coast of Asia

from Siberia to New Zealand. Twenty percent of these volcanoes

are located in Indonesia. Other big groupings are in Japan,

the Aleutian Islands, and Central America.

In May nineteen eighty, Mount Saint Helens blew its top

in Washington State.

The huge explosion came as a great surprise to geologists.

They'd measured the Cascade Mountain Range for several decades.

But they hadn't expected so much destruction.

The eruption of Mount St. Helens sent hot volcanic ash and gases

into the air. It caused severe mud slides and avalanches.

It killed trees, crops, animals, and people.

It damaged roads, buildings, and bridges.

Fortunately, not everything was lost:

wheat and apples grew very well in the volcanic ash.

Listen to your recording.

Did you make the key word in each phrase higher and longer than the other words in each phrase?

Did you make the content words longer and clearer than the function words?

Did you say the correct number of syllables?

Did you stress the correct syllable in each word?

Did you pronounce the sounds /ʃ/ and /ʒ/ clearly?

Did you pronounce the sounds /tʃ/ and /dʒ/ clearly?

Did you make a clear difference between /ʃ/ and /tʃ/?

Did you make a clear difference between /ʒ/ and /dʒ/?

In which of these areas do you need to improve?

In what other areas do you need to improve?

TOPICS FOR ORAL OR WRITTEN COMPOSITION

1. Explain how a volcano erupts. Discuss the geological conditions which cause lava, steam, and ashes to be thrown out through the earth's crust (surface).

2. Describe the eruption of Mount St. Helens (or another volcano). Give more details than were presented in this lesson.

3. Choose and tell about one aspect studied by a particular kind of scientist, such as a biologist, meteorologist, archeologist, anthropologist, linguist, physicist, etc.

Chapter 13

Father's Idea of Fun

VOCABULARY FOCUS

Do you or your classmates know the words in this list? Complete each sentence with a word or phrase from the list. Change nouns and verbs to appropriate forms. Discuss your choices with a partner.

agreeable	chuckle	fold	plant
anyway	dive	gopher	poke
benevolent	drag	grip	stroll
chat	familiar	Mother Nature	tug
cheerfully		old fogy	

1. Fred _____ the letter and put it into an envelope.

2. Be careful how you carry your umbrella or you might _____ somebody with it.

3. Jeff _____ on the knot until it finally came loose.

4. "I'm having a lot of fun!" Vivian exclaimed _____.

5. A _____ is a type of ratlike animal that makes holes in the ground and lives in them.

6. "Haven't we met before? Your face looks so

_____ to me."

7. Ophelia climbed onto a rock and _____ into

the lake with a big splash.

8. Today's weather is neither too hot nor too cold; it's quite

_____.

9. An _____ is a person who has old-fashioned

habits and dislikes change.

10. People can control some aspects of their lives, but other aspects

are controlled by _____.

11. The desk was too heavy to lift, so they _____

it across the room.

12. The cat _____ itself in the sunshine by the

window and refused to leave until the sun moved.

13. The child had taken such a firm _____ on the

dog's tail that it couldn't run away.

14. When Vincent got together with his friends, they sat and

_____ about old times.

15. Everyone thought the joke was funny. Some

_____ quietly, while others laughed loudly.

16. *"A Ghostly Adventure"* was a scary movie; that's what I think,

_____.

17. Giving money to needy people is a _____ act.

18. After having a heavy meal, Victoria likes to take a short

_____ to help digest her food.

BEFORE YOU LISTEN

Look at the picture and tell what you think.

How old is the boy?
What are the two men doing?
What are the relationships among the three people?

Victor is an active young boy who loves to run and play outdoors. His father, on the other hand, prefers to stroll leisurely. When the two of them go on a walk together, their differences are sure to appear.

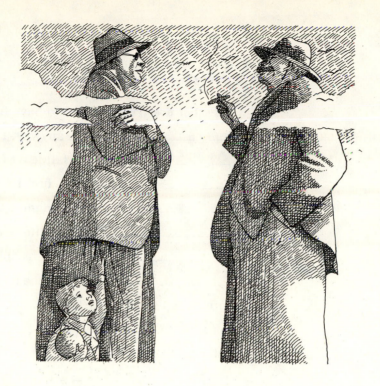

LISTENING COMPREHENSION

Read these statements. Listen to the passage and choose the best answer for each statement.

1. Victor thinks _____ is fun.
   - a. feeding dogs
   - b. fighting dogs
   - c. fitting docks
   - d. feeding ducks

2. Victor's father _____ suggests going for a walk.
   - a. always
   - b. usually
   - c. sometimes
   - d. seldom

3. Victor is interested in _____.
   - a. walking with his father
   - b. catching frogs
   - c. going downtown
   - d. chuckling

4. Whenever Victor's father wants to stop, Victor _____.
   - a. has to stop
   - b. wants to stop
   - c. plants his feet stiffly
   - d. chats with old fogies.

5. Victor pokes his finger into his father's _____
   - a. pants
   - b. hand
   - c. thigh
   - d. tie

6. The father seems to be _____ by Victor's behavior.
   - a. amused
   - b. worried
   - c. excited
   - d. upset

7. Victor doesn't feel _____ taking a walk with his father.
   - a. bored
   - b. powerless
   - c. small
   - d. satisfied

LISTENING CLOZE

Listen to the passage again. Fill in the words you hear, one word for each blank. Pause the tape as necessary.

Father doesn't know how to have fun, not in my

(1) _____, anyway. I think jumping

(2) _____ fall leaves or playing ball in the

(3) _____ is fun. He thinks

(4) _____ undignified for a fellow his

(5) _____. I think feeding

(6) _____ is agreeable

(7) _____, but he says to leave that job to Mother

Nature. Every so often, he'll say (8) _____, "Let's

go for a walk, Victor." Then he (9) _____ me

downtown. Whenever he wants to stop, I have to stop, too. He folds his

arms, (10) _____ his feet stiffly, and

chats forever with other old (11) _____. I tug on his

pants or (12) _____ my finger into his

(13) _____, but Father simply smiles down

(14) _____ me from the clouds. If a

(15) _____ jumps across the road or a gopher pops

(16) _____ head out of a hole, I'll

(17) _____ toward it. I never get far before feeling

Father's (18) _____ grip on me, gentle but very

firm. Then he (19) _____ and gives me a

(20) _____ pat on the back. Taking a walk with

him is not my idea of having fun.

DISCUSSION

How does Victor like to have fun?

Why does Victor tug on his father's pants and poke his finger into his thigh?

Do you sympathize (share feelings) more with Victor or with his father?

SOUND FOCUS 1: /f/

To produce the sound /f/, as in *fall,* place your upper front teeth loosely on your lower lip. Let your voiceless breath flow out continuously and smoothly between the center of your lower lip and your upper teeth.[1]

Underline the letters that make /f/ sound in the following words.

fall	leaf	cheerful	from
fun	laugh	gopher	frog
field	cliff	dignified	fly
photo	enough	stiffly	raft

SOUND FOCUS 2: /v/

To produce the sound /v/, as in _very_, place your upper front teeth on your lower lip as for /f/. This time, let out a continuous voiced sound.

very	leave	every	advice
view	have	having	curved
Victor	dive	forever	behaved
volcano	give	benevolent	convenient

SOUND FOCUS 3: VOWEL LENGTH

A. Hold the vowel longer when it comes before the voiced /v/ sound.

_/-f/_	_/—v/_
leaf	l ea ve
safe	s a ve
half	h a ve
proof	pr o ve

B. Underline the long vowels in the following sentences. Then practice saying them, paying attention to vowel length.

A leaf dropped into the food.
Leave the pot of rice on the stove.
Rise before the sun reaches this side.
Pat took five baths in one evening.
I'll have the big half and give you the small half.
When a baby teethes, she cries a lot.
Bev washed the garage roof.
Frank watched them fix the bridge.

---

[1]To check yourself, place your hand in front of your mouth and feel the continuous flow of air. If you hold a small piece of paper in front of your mouth, it will move continuously, though not as much as for /θ/.

SOUND FOCUS 4: INTRODUCTORY PHRASE INTONATION

A. Review rising ↗ and falling ↘ intonation. Listen to these mini-dialogs and mark the final intonation. Then practice with a partner.

1	2
A: Dinner? ↗	*A:* Now.
B: Sounds good. ↘	*B:* Now?
A: Next Friday?	*A:* Yes. Together.
B: Sure.	*B:* Together?
A: Six-thirty?	*A:* Right.
B: Seven.	*B:* By bus?
	A: By car. Okay?
	B: Okay.

B. When a phrase or clause comes before the main clause of a sentence, there is usually a slight rise at the end of the first phrase. This rising intonation indicates that the speaker has not yet finished the sentence.

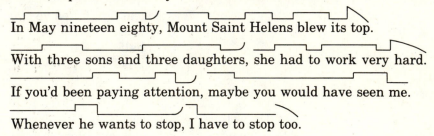

In May nineteen eighty, Mount Saint Helens blew its top.

With three sons and three daughters, she had to work very hard.

If you'd been paying attention, maybe you would have seen me.

Whenever he wants to stop, I have to stop too.

C. Practice saying these sentences to a partner, rising slightly at the end of the introductory phrase.

> Every so often, he'll invite me for a walk.
> If a gopher pops its head out of a hole, I'll dive toward it.
> This evening, I'm going to practice stress and intonation.
> After I've practiced, I'll sound a lot more natural.

SOUND FOCUS 5: CONTRASTIVE STRESS AND INTONATION

A. From the previous lessons, you know that *function words,* (such as personal pronouns, articles, conjunctions and auxiliary verbs) are usually *unstressed;* that is, they are weak, short, reduced, and low. On the other hand, *content words* are generally *stressed,* and the *last* content word is usually stressed more than any other word in a phrase. Listen to these sentences spoken with normal phrase stress.

I gave her the móney.

Mary and John can gó.

The book is on the désk.

Did you buy a récord?

Did you see them in the óffice?

B. However, to show emphasis or contrast, any word the speaker considers important may be stressed, including function words. Listen to the words that are contrasted. They are louder, longer, clearer, and higher than the others.

Í gave her the money. Yóu didn't give it to her.
I gave hér the money. I didn't give it to hím.
I gáve her the money. I didn't lénd it to her.

He didn't say Mary and John cóuld go. He said they cóuldn't go.
He didn't say Mary ór John could go. He said Mary ánd John could go.
He didn't sáy Mary and John could go. He implíed they could go.

The book is ón the desk. It isn't ín the desk.
The book ís on the desk. I pút it there just a mínute ago.

Did you búy a record or bórrow one?
Did yóu buy a record or did someone élse buy one?
Did you buy á record or sóme records?[2]

Did yóu see them in the office or did shé see them there?
Did you sée them in the office or did you see ús there?
Did you see them ín the office or outsíde the office?

C. Mark the phrase stress in the following sentences. For the first sentence, use normal phrase stress. For the next, use contrastive stress. Then practice saying them to a partner.

I know you want to go.
I know you want to go, but you can't.
I know you want to go, but I don't.

These are their tickets.
These are their tickets, not ours.
These are their tickets, not those.

---

[2]Note that "a" is pronounced /ə/ when unstressed, but /eʸ/ when stressed, as in this sentence.

That isn't my coat.
That isn't my coat. I think it's yours.
That isn't my coat. This is mine.

He doesn't like horses.
He doesn't like horses, but I do.
He doesn't like horses, but he takes care of them.

Do they want me to see you?
Do they want me to see you or him?
Do they want me to see you or does he want me to see you?

I'm flying from San Francisco.
I'm flying from San Francisco. I'm not driving.
I'm flying from San Francisco, not to San Francisco.

Is that a photograph of Liz?
Is that a photograph of Liz or for Liz?
Is that a photograph of Liz, or isn't it?

SOUNDS IN CONTEXT: PHRASE BY PHRASE 1

Listen and mark the phrase stress. Then rewind the tape and practice the passage in short phrases.

Fáther doesn't know | how to have fún, | not in mý view, |
anyway. | I think | jumping in fall leaves | or playing ball in the field |
is fun. | He thinks | it's undignified | for a fellow his age. | I think |
feeding ducks is agreeable enough, | but he says | to leave that job |
to Mother Nature. | Every so often, | he'll say cheerfully, |
"Let's go for a walk, | Victor." | Then he drags me | downtown. |
Whenever he wants to stop, | I have to stop, | too. | He folds his arms, |
plants his feet stiffly, | and chats forever | with other old fogies. |
I tug on his pants | or poke my finger | into his thigh, |
but Father simply smiles down at me | from the clouds. |
If a frog jumps across the road | or a gopher pops its head out of a hole, |
I'll dive toward it. | I never get far |
before feeling Father's familiar grip on me, | gentle | but very firm. |
Then he chuckles | and gives me a benevolent pat | on the back. |
Taking a walk with him | is not my idea | of having fun. |

SOUNDS IN CONTEXT: PHRASE BY PHRASE 2

Listen and underline the /f/ sounds once and the /v/ sounds twice. (Note that /f/ sounds can be written with **f, gh,** and **ph,** and /v/ sounds with **v** and **f.**) Then rewind the tape and practice the passage in longer phrases.

Father doesn't know how to ha<u>ve</u> fun, | not in my <u>v</u>iew, anyway. |
I think jumping in fall leaves | or playing ball in the field | is fun. |
He thinks it's undignified | for a fellow his age. |
I think feeding ducks is agreeable enough, |
but he says to leave that job to Mother Nature. |
Every so often, he'll say cheerfully, | "Let's go for a walk, Victor." |
Then he drags me downtown. | Whenever he wants to stop, |
I have to stop, too. | He folds his arms, plants his feet stiffly, |
and chats forever with other old fogies. | I tug on his pants |
or poke my finger into his thigh, |
but Father simply smiles down at me from the clouds. |
If a frog jumps across the road | or a gopher pops its head out of a hole, |
I'll dive toward it. | I never get far |
before feeling Father's familiar grip on me, | gentle but very firm. |
Then he chuckles | and gives me a benevolent pat on the back. |
Taking a walk with him | is not my idea of having fun. |

SOUNDS IN CONTEXT: PHRASE BY PHRASE 3

Listen and cross out the unstressed words. Then rewind the tape and practice the passage in complete sentences. As you speak, clap out the rhythm with your hands.

Father doesn't know how ~~to~~ have fun, not ~~in~~ my view, anyway. |
I think jumping in fall leaves or playing ball in the field is fun. |
He thinks it's undignified for a fellow his age. | I think feeding ducks
is agreeable enough, but he says to leave that job to Mother Nature. |
Every so often, he'll say cheerfully, "Let's go for a walk, Victor." |
Then he drags me downtown. | Whenever he wants to stop,
I have to stop, too. | He folds his arms, plants his feet stiffly,
and chats forever with other old fogies. |
I tug on his pants or poke my finger into his thigh,
but Father simply smiles down at me from the clouds. |
If a frog jumps across the road or a gopher pops its head out of a hole,
I'll dive toward it. | I never get far before
feeling Father's familiar grip on me, gentle but very firm. |
Then he chuckles and gives me a benevolent pat on the back. |
Taking a walk with him is not my idea of having fun. |

ON YOUR OWN

Review the **Sound Focus** exercises introduced in this lesson.
Practice **Phrase by Phrase** steps several times.
Record the passage from beginning to end without stopping.

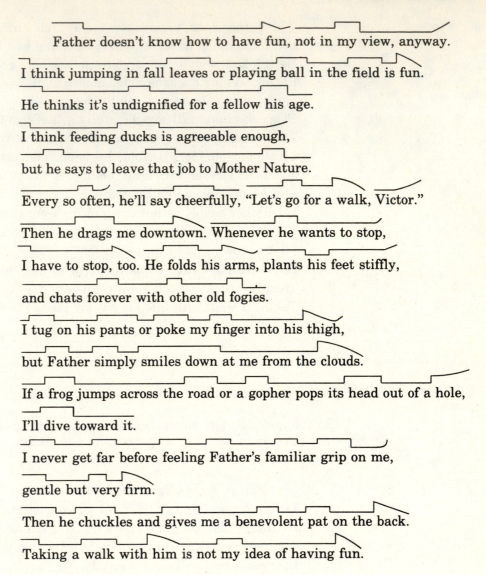

Father doesn't know how to have fun, not in my view, anyway.

I think jumping in fall leaves or playing ball in the field is fun.

He thinks it's undignified for a fellow his age.

I think feeding ducks is agreeable enough,

but he says to leave that job to Mother Nature.

Every so often, he'll say cheerfully, "Let's go for a walk, Victor."

Then he drags me downtown. Whenever he wants to stop,

I have to stop, too. He folds his arms, plants his feet stiffly,

and chats forever with other old fogies.

I tug on his pants or poke my finger into his thigh,

but Father simply smiles down at me from the clouds.

If a frog jumps across the road or a gopher pops its head out of a hole,

I'll dive toward it.

I never get far before feeling Father's familiar grip on me,

gentle but very firm.

Then he chuckles and gives me a benevolent pat on the back.

Taking a walk with him is not my idea of having fun.

Listen to your recording.

Did you say words together in thought phrases?

Did you make the key words in each phrase stronger and higher than the other words?

Did you make a distinction between clear and reduced vowels?

Did you lengthen vowels followed by voiced consonants?

Did you practice consonant-to-vowel, vowel-to-consonant, vowel-to-vowel linking and consonant-to-consonant holding?

Did you pronounce the sounds /f/ and /v/ clearly?

In which of these areas do you need to improve?

In what other areas do you need to improve?

TOPICS FOR ORAL OR WRITTEN COMPOSITION

1. Have you ever had an experience like this young boy's? Were you and your father (or mother) interested in different things? How did you behave?

2. The term *generation gap* refers to the wide difference between the viewpoints or tastes of one generation and those of another. Do you feel a generation gap between you (or your generation) and your parents (or their generation)? Give one or two examples of the ways you differ greatly.

3. Contrast how you and a friend do the same task, for example: cook, study, drive, or travel. Describe the differences in the way the two of you try to reach the same goal.

Chapter 14

Edison's Creative Talent

VOCABULARY FOCUS

Do you or your classmates know the words in this list? Complete each sentence with a word or phrase from the list. Change nouns and verbs to appropriate forms. Discuss your choices with a partner.

analyze	inspiration	patent	recognize
creative	kinetoscope	perspiration	relationship
concept	modest	phonograph	talent
device	motion picture	process	youth
genius			

1. A _____ person produces original ideas and things.

2. A _____ is special natural ability or skill.

3. A _____ is a piece of writing from a government office (Patent Office). It gives someone the right to make or sell a new invention for a certain number of years.

4. A _____ is a person who has very special intellectual or creative power.

5. A _____ is the series of actions or changes that leads to a result. It is the manner in which something happens.

6. To examine something carefully in order to find out about it is to _____ it.

7. A _____ is a general thought, idea, or understanding.

8. A _____ is an instrument, especially one that is cleverly thought out.

9. A movie, or a film, can also be called a _____.

10. If two things or people are connected, or if they are similar, we can say there is a _____ between them.

11. People all over the world consider Thomas Edison a great inventor. He is _____ as a great inventor.

12. When people comment that she is successful, and she says that it's just because she had good luck, she's being _____.

13. _____ is the early period of life when a person is young.

14. _____ is something (or someone) that makes a person want to produce good and beautiful things.

15. Liquid that comes out from the body through the skin to cool it is called sweat, or _____.

16. A _____ is an instrument which can play the music or sounds of a record. It is also called a record player.

17. A _____ was an early motion-picture machine. It had film that wound back and forth on rollers, allowing a person to see moving images through a tiny hole in the top of the large machine.

BEFORE YOU LISTEN

Look at the picture and tell what you think.

Edison is looking through a kinetoscope. What does he see?
Are there several horses or just one horse?

Thomas Alva Edison (1847–1931) was an American who invented many devices in such fields as telegraphy, phonography, electric lighting, and photography. He obtained more patents than any other inventor in the United States. His inventions have helped change the world we live in. Can you name any of his inventions?

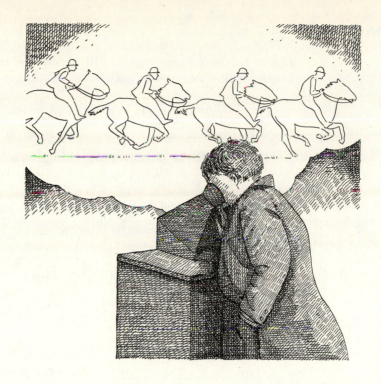

LISTENING COMPREHENSION

Read these statements. Listen to the passage and choose the best answer for each statement.

1. Thomas Edison started inventing things in his old age. _____
   a. True   b. False   c. We can't tell

2. The light bulb is one of his inventions. _____
   a. True   b. False   c. We can't tell

3. Motion pictures developed from the kinetoscope that Edison invented. _____
   a. True   b. False   c. We can't tell

4. Edison made 10,000 inventions. _____
   a. True   b. False   c. We can't tell

5. Edison said, "Genius is . . . _____ percent perspiration."
   a. ninety-five   b. nineteen   c. ninety-nine

6. Edison's papers tell about his _____.
   a. death   b. relationships c. creative process

7. Edison saw relationships between things that _____ related.
   a. were   b. seemed   c. didn't seem

8. _____ of us are as talented as Edison.
   a. Most   b. A few   c. Few

LISTENING CLOZE

Listen to the passage again. Fill in the words you hear, one word for each blank. Pause the tape as necessary.

Thomas Edison is recognized as one of the

(1) _____ greatest (2) _____ .

This genius began inventing things as a (3) _____

and kept on until old (4) _____ . He invented the

phonograph and the light (5) _____ , now common

devices. His kinetoscope later (6) _____ to motion

pictures. These are just (7) _____ few of his eleven

hundred inventions. But Edison said (8) _____ ,

"Genius is one percent inspiration and ninety-nine percent

(9) _____ ."

Many people think there's a lot more to it than

(10) _____ . After his

(11) _____ , millions of Edison's papers

(12) _____ found. They tell a lot about his

inventions and his (13) _____ process. He saw

relationships between things that didn't seem

(14) _____ . For example, he showed that the ear

could (15) _____ sound from a phonograph. Then

he analyzed that the (16) _____ , in the same way,

could see pictures (17) _____ a kinetoscope. This

(18) _____ is hard for most of us to understand, for

(19) _____ of us are (20) _____

talented as Edison!

DISCUSSION

What did Edison mean by "Genius is one percent inspiration and ninety-nine percent perspiration?" Do you agree?

Do many people understand how Edison developed his concepts into inventions?

Which of Edison's inventions do you appreciate the most?

SOUND FOCUS 1: /eʸ/

To produce the sound /eʸ/, as in _say,_ raise the front part of your tongue to a central position in your mouth. Keep the tip of your tongue low and relaxed. It may touch the back of your lower teeth. As you make a voiced sound, glide the middle of your tongue forward and upward toward the position of the sound /i/. At the same time, pull the corners of your lips back.

Underline the letters that make the sound /eʸ/. Draw a slash (/) through the reduced, or schwa, vowels.

s<u>ay</u>	great∅st	related
same	later	relationships
rain	papers	inspiration
take	creative	perspiration

SOUND FOCUS 2: /ɛ/

To produce the sound /ɛ/, as in _every,_ raise the front part of your tongue to a central position, slightly lower than for the sound /eʸ/. Keep your tongue low and relaxed. As you make a voiced sound, do not let your tongue glide.

Underline the letters that make the sound /ɛ/. Draw a slash (/) through the reduced vowels.

<u>e</u>v∅ry	<u>E</u>dis∅n	kinetoscope
led	recognize	eleven
death	inventors	percent
said	many	concept

SOUND FOCUS 3: /æ/

To produce the sound /æ/, as in _act,_ lower your jaw and tongue slightly more than for /eʸ/ or /ɛ/. Keep the tip of your tongue low and relaxed. Push the front part of your tongue slightly forward. Make a voiced sound. At the same time, pull the corners of your lips back. Do not let your tongue glide.

Underline the letters that make the sound /æ/. Draw a slash (/) through the reduced vowels.

<u>a</u>ct	example	talented
cat	analyze	actually
laugh	analysis	phonograph
pack	understand	capacity

SOUND FOCUS 4: SOUND AND STRESS SHIFTS

A. Listen to the sound and stress shifts in the following word families. Draw the intonation line.

telescope   telescópic   telescópically

microscope   microscopic   microscopically

kinetoscope   kinetoscopic

educate   education   educated

populate   population   populated

generate   generation   generated

inspire   inspiration   inspirational   inspirationally

perspire   perspiration

converse   conversation   conversational   conversationally

repeat   repetition   repetitive   repetitively

define   definition   definitive   definitively

compete   competition   competitive   competitively

photograph   photography   photographer   photographic   photographically

phonograph   phonography   phonographer   phonographic   phonographically

telegraph   telegraphy   telegrapher   telegraphic   telegraphically

B. Take turns saying these words to a partner, marking the syllables and word stress. Use the stress shift patterns you've studied in this and the previous lesson as a guide.

illustrate, illustration   educational, educated

graduation, graduated   recognize, recognition

contribution, contribute   cooperate, cooperation

communicate, communication   combination, combine

geographically, geographer   orthographic, orthography

biographer, biography   autobiography, autobiographical

compete, competitive   exclude, exclusively

SOUND FOCUS 5: CONTRASTIVE STRESS AND INTONATION

A few multisyllabic word pairs differ by only one syllable. To make a contrast between them, the word stress changes to the syllable that differentiates them. Listen to the following sentences and mark the stress. Normal word and phrase stress is used in the first sentence, and contrastive stress is used in the following sentence(s).

I'm encouraged.

Did you say encouraged or discouraged?

Let's eat our lunch outside.

It's a bit windy outside. Why don't we eat inside today?

She said to meet at ten-thirty.

You mean she changed it from nine-thirty to ten-thirty?

Sixteen recordings have been handed in.

Why are there only sixteen recordings when there are nineteen students?

I wonder where Edison got his inspiration.

He said that genius is one percent inspiration and ninety-nine percent perspiration.

Our school just ordered some new lenses.

The biology department needed microscopic lenses and the astronomy department needed telescopic lenses.

SOUNDS IN CONTEXT: PHRASE BY PHRASE 1

Listen and mark the stressed syllables with (ˊ) and the unstressed syllables with (·). Then rewind the tape and practice the passage in short phrases.

Thomas Edison | is recognized | as one of the world's | greatest inventors. | This genius | began inventing things | as a youth | and kept on until old age. | He invented the phonograph |

and the light bulb, | now common devices. | His kinetoscope |
later led to motion pictures. | These are just a few of his eleven
hundred inventions. | But Edison said modestly, |
"Genius | is one percent inspiration | and ninety-nine percent |
perspiration." |

      Many people think | there's a lot more to it | than that. |
After his death, | millions of Edison's papers | were found. |
They tell a lot | about his inventions | and his creative process. |
He saw relationships | between things | that did not seem related. |
For example, | he showed that the ear | could hear sound |
from a phonograph. | Then he analyzed | that the eye, |
in the same way, | could see pictures | through a kinetoscope. |
This concept is hard | for most of us to understand, | for few of us |
are as talented as Edison! |

SOUNDS IN CONTEXT: PHRASE BY PHRASE 2

Listen and underline the /eʸ/ sounds. Draw a slash (/) through the reduced /ə/
(schwa) vowels. (Note that the sound /eʸ/ can be written with **a, ai, ay,** and **ea.**)
Then rewind the tape and practice the passage in longer phrases.

      Thom/as Edis/on is rec/ognized |
/as one /of th/e world's great/est invent/ors. |
This genius began inventing things as a youth |
and kept on until old age. |
He invented the phonograph and the light bulb, | now common devices. |
His kinetoscope later led to motion pictures. |
These are just a few | of his eleven hundred inventions. |
But Edison said modestly, | "Genius is one percent inspiration |
and ninety-nine percent perspiration." |
      Many people think | there's a lot more to it than that. |
After his death, | millions of Edison's papers were found. |
They tell a lot about his inventions | and his creative process. |
He saw relationships | between things that did not seem related. |
For example, |
he showed that the ear could hear sound from a phonograph. |
Then he analyzed that the eye, in the same way, |
could see pictures through a kinetoscope. |
This concept is hard for most of us to understand, |
for few of us are as talented as Edison! |

SOUNDS IN CONTEXT: PHRASE BY PHRASE 3

Listen and underline the /ɛ/ sounds once and the /æ/ sounds twice. (Note that the sound /ɛ/ can be written with **e, ea, ai,** and **a,** and the sound /æ/ with **a and au.**) Then rewind the tape and practice the passage in complete sentences.

Thomas Edison is recognized as one of the world's greatest
inventors. | This genius began inventing things as a youth and kept on
until old age. | He invented the phonograph and the light bulb,
now common devices. | His kinetoscope later led to motion pictures. |
These are just a few of his eleven hundred inventions. |
But Edison said modestly, "Genius is one percent inspiration
and ninety-nine percent perspiration." |
Many people think there's a lot more to it than that. |
After his death, millions of Edison's papers were found. |
They tell a lot about his inventions and his creative process. |
He saw relationships between things that did not seem related. |
For example, he showed that the ear could hear sound from a phonograph. |
Then he analyzed that the eye, in the same way,
could see pictures through a kinetoscope. |
This concept is hard for most of us to understand,
for few of us are as talented as Edison! |

ON YOUR OWN

Review the **Sound Focus** exercises introduced in this lesson.
Practice **Phrase by Phrase** steps several times.
Record the passage from beginning to end without stopping.

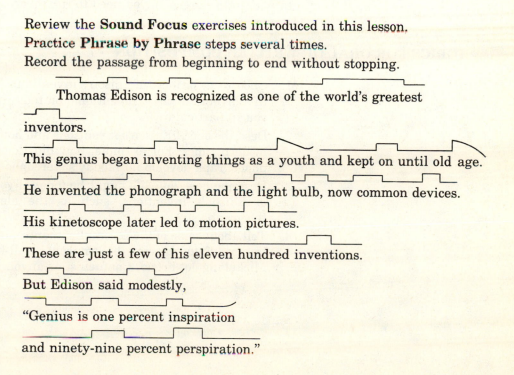

Thomas Edison is recognized as one of the world's greatest
inventors.

This genius began inventing things as a youth and kept on until old age.

He invented the phonograph and the light bulb, now common devices.

His kinetoscope later led to motion pictures.

These are just a few of his eleven hundred inventions.

But Edison said modestly,

"Genius is one percent inspiration

and ninety-nine percent perspiration."

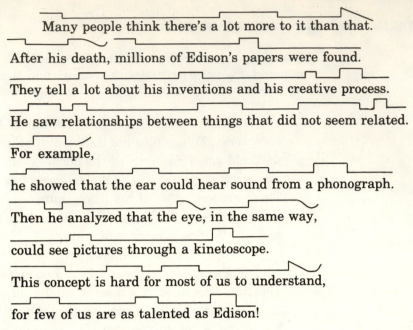

Many people think there's a lot more to it than that.

After his death, millions of Edison's papers were found.

They tell a lot about his inventions and his creative process.

He saw relationships between things that did not seem related.

For example,

he showed that the ear could hear sound from a phonograph.

Then he analyzed that the eye, in the same way,

could see pictures through a kinetoscope.

This concept is hard for most of us to understand,

for few of us are as talented as Edison!

Listen to your recording.

Did you say the correct number of syllables?

Did you stress the correct syllable in each word?

Did you say the key word of each phrase longer and higher?

Did you make a distinction between clear and reduced vowels?

Did you pronounce the sounds /e^y/, /ɛ/, and /æ/ clearly?

Did you practice consonant-to-vowel, vowel-to-consonant, vowel-to-vowel linking and consonant-to-consonant holding?

In which of these areas do you need to improve?

In what other areas do you need to improve?

TOPICS FOR ORAL OR WRITTEN COMPOSITION

1. Choose one or more of Edison's inventions. Discuss the importance of this invention (these inventions) on today's society in general, or on you in particular.

2. Describe one of Edison's inventions and how it has advanced through modern times. For example, how did Edison's early hand-operated phonograph develop into today's stereophonic electric record player?

3. Describe how your life might be today if you did not have use of one of Edison's inventions, such as the electric light bulb or the telegraph.

4. Tell about some of the accomplishments of an inventor or a specialist in any field. It may be someone well-known, such as Mozart, Michelangelo, Freud, Confucius, or anyone else you admire.

Chapter 15

Baby Boomers: The Big Bulge

VOCABULARY FOCUS

Do you or your classmates know the words in this list? Complete each sentence with a word or phrase from the list. Change nouns and verbs to appropriate forms. Discuss your choices with a partner.

boom	flexible	labor force
bulge	flood	outnumber
computer literate	generation	polio
consumer	have an edge on	postwar
consumer goods	impact	threat
depression	independent	vie
diphtheria		

1. My parents, my children and I represent three
    _____.

2. If there are more women than men, we can say that women
    _____ men.

3. The _____ means the group of people in
    society who work for wages.

4. A _____ is someone who buys and uses goods
    and services.

5. Goods such as clothing and appliances, which people buy and use
    for personal needs or desires, are called _____.

6. A _____ is a rapid growth or increase. It is also the noise from an explosion.

7. Someone who does not need things or other people is _____. He or she is self-reliant or self-determined.

8. Someone or something that can change to be suitable for new needs or changed conditions is _____.

9. A person who is able to understand and/or use computers is _____.

10. An _____ is a shocking effect or impression.

11. The time after a war can be called the _____

12. A _____ is a period of extremely reduced business activity and high unemployment.

13. To arrive somewhere in large numbers, usually too many at once, is to _____ that place.

14. If you have an advantage over someone (or something) else, you _____ that person or situation.

15. To _____ for something means to compete or to struggle for it.

16. Pressure can cause something to swell and make a _____ in the surface.

17. A _____ is a warning of coming hurt, pain, or danger.

18. _____ is a serious infectious disease of the throat which makes breathing difficult.

19. _____ is a serious infectious disease of the spine (nerves in the backbone), often resulting in paralysis (a lasting loss of the power to move certain muscles).

BEFORE YOU LISTEN

Look at the picture and tell what you think.

What is the difference in the shape of the two buildings?
Why is the one on the left bulging?
Are the people going to work, to study, to play, to rest?

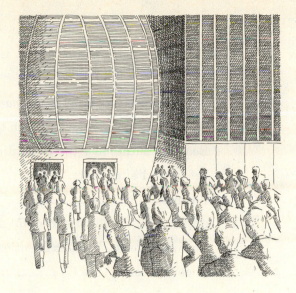

The number of American babies born during the Depression of the 1930s and World War II (1939–1945) was very low. After the war, from 1946 to 1964, the number of babies born increased rapidly. This generation is known as the Baby Boom.

LISTENING COMPREHENSION

Read these statements. Listen to the passage and choose the best answer for each statement.

1. The Baby Boom population is bigger than their children's generation.

    _____

    a. True   b. False   c. We can't tell

2. Baby Boomers flooded the labor force in the 1920s and 1930s. _____
    a. True   b. False   c. We can't tell

3. The competition for jobs among Baby Boomers is very rough. _____
    a. True   b. False   c. We can't tell

4. Baby Boomers are better off than their parents in some ways.

    _____

    a. True   b. False   c. We can't tell

5. Diptheria and polio were more common diseases among Baby Boomers than among their parents. _____
    a. True   b. False   c. We can't tell

6. The number of college graduates among Baby Boomers is nearly double the number of college graduates among their parents' generation. _____
    a. True   b. False   c. We can't tell

7. Baby Boomers get married later than their parents did. _____
    a. True   b. False   c. We can't tell

LISTENING CLOZE

Listen to the passage again. Fill in the words you hear, one word for each blank. Pause the tape as necessary.

The postwar Baby Boom has made a very big

(1) _____ on the American population. Baby

Boomers outnumber the generations (2) _____

before and after them. In (3) _____ youth, Baby

Boomers (4) _____ new schools to open. Growing

up, they required more food, (5) _____, and

consumer goods. In their twenties and (6) _____,

Boomers flooded the (7) _____ force. Finding more

people than ever (8) _____ for the same position,

they (9) _____ big problems in employment. In

some ways, Baby Boomers are better (10) _____

than their parents. For example, Boomers grew up with little

(11) _____ of diphtheria and

(12) _____. One-fourth are college graduates,

almost twice as many as their (13) _____.

Computer (14) _____ Boomers have an

(15) _____ on older workers. Most Baby Boom

women, more (16) _____ than their mothers, work

outside the home. Baby Boomers tend to be more flexible and

(17) _____. They marry later and have

(18) _____ children. Baby Boomers have changed

(19) _____ in many ways, and will continue

(20) _____ for a long time.

DISCUSSION

In what way does the Baby Boom generation represent a bulge?
How has the Baby Boom generation made such a big impact on American society?
Name several ways Baby Boomers are better off than their parents.
Are Baby Boomers worse off in any ways?

SOUND FOCUS 1: /p/

A. To produce the sound /p/, as in *people,* press your lips together tightly. This stops the air from flowing out of your mouth. Let your voiceless breath blow against your lips, forcing them to open sharply. When the sound /p/ comes before a vowel in a stressed syllable, release a sharp and strong puff of air as for the voiceless stops /t/ and /k/.[1]

Underline the letters that make the /p/ sound.

pay	parents	appear
pan	polio	repay
push	people	computer
paper	popular	independent

B. When the sound /p/ comes at the end of a phrase, do not separate your lips. When the sound /p/ comes at the beginning of an unstressed syllable, at the end of a syllable that is not linked to the next syllable, or after the sound /s/, do not release a puff of air.

up	napkin	speak
top	stopping	spell
cap	open	especially
hopeless	upper	spray

SOUND FOCUS 2: /b/

To produce the sound /b/, as in *baby*, press your lips together tightly, as for the sound /p/. Blow against your lips, forcing them to open sharply, but make a voiced sound. Like other stop sounds, /b/ is not released at the end of a syllable that is not linked to the following sound.

Underline the letters that make the /b/ sound.

big	better	lab	labor
baby	about	cub	double
boom	began	rib	outnumber
both	before	bulb	brave

SOUND FOCUS 3: VOWEL LENGTH

A. The first word in each pair below ends in a voiceless /p/. The second word ends in a voiced /b/. Hold the vowel longer when it is followed by a voiced sound.

/-p/	/—b/
rope —	r o be
nap —	n a b
cap —	c a b
rip —	r i b

---

[1]Test yourself by placing a piece of paper in front of your mouth. It should move suddenly as you pronounce the sound /p/ with a puff of air.

B. Practice saying these sentences to a partner, completing each sentence with one of the *italicized* words. Have your partner raise one finger if the first word was heard, and two fingers if the second was heard.

1. I bought a *rope/robe*.
2. I need a *cap/cab*.
3. There's a *rip/rib*.
4. Put the *rack/rag* in the back.
5. The *wick/wig* is wet.
6. I saw some *ice/eyes*.
7. She *wrote/rode* it.
8. When is *March/Marge* coming?
9. Give him a *cart/card*.
10. Say the word *"teeth"/"teethe"*.

SOUND FOCUS 4: NOUN COMPOUND REVIEW

The main stress of a noun compound is on the first word of the compound.

Adjective + Noun	*Noun Compound*
Liz's óffice	póst office
old friénd	gírlfriend
foreign lánguage	sígn language

A. Listen to each of the following phrases and mark the stress. If it is a noun compound, put a check (√) in the blank.

1. parking lot	√	7. math department	_____
2. Baby Boom	_____	8. waterfall	_____
3. perfect master	_____	9. volcanic ash	_____
4. many ways	_____	10. mountain range	_____
5. labor force	_____	11. train station	_____
6. flower boxes	_____	12. hiking boots	_____

B. Take turns saying these sentences to a partner, paying attention to *Adjective + Noun* phrases and *Noun Compounds*. Have your partner listen for good stress and intonation.

1. They have three daughters in the work force.
2. The teenagers started a new exercise program.
3. I saw my English teacher in the parking lot.

4.   He mailed a money order at the post office.

5.   A baby sitter looked after my baby sister.

6.   Let's get some ice cream and candy bars.

7.   Has the Baby Boom changed American society?

8.   Would you buy four light bulbs at the supermarket?

9.   Did he meet his girlfriend at the airport or the train station?

10.   Is your mother a fire fighter or a police officer?

11.   They took their hiking boots, swimsuits, and fishing rods.

12.   Do you have a headache, a stomach ache or a backache?

SOUND FOCUS 5: CONSONANT REVIEW

Practice saying these sentences to a partner. Pay particular attention to the consonant sounds. Stress the content words.

1.   Patty put her book and pen in her bag.

2.   The bank in Berkeley was robbed yesterday evening.

3.   Fay bought a very fine pair of brown boots.

4.   Victor put the telephone on the far table in the bedroom.

5.   Purple and blue are Bobbie's favorite colors.

6.   Some of Nan's friends sang songs for Bob and Mom and Pop.

7.   Why is Ralph wearing his red hat and vest?

8.   Helen and Fannie saw five huge fish with very big fins.

9.   We have thousands of visitors from France these days.

10.   We took them to see the zebras in the zoo.

11.   Lynn's neighbor likes to take long naps during the day.

12.   Dolly Jones looked pretty worried yesterday.

13.   Sheila says Elizabeth should sell chairs.

14.   Zena chose a yellow jacket and yellow shoes.

15.   Curtis put a long log against the back gate.

SOUNDS IN CONTEXT: PHRASE BY PHRASE 1

Listen and mark the stressed syllables with (ˊ) and the unstressed syllables with (·). Then rewind the tape and practice the passage in short phrases. While you speak, clap out the rhythm.

The postwar Baby Boom | has made a very big impact |
on the American population. | Baby Boomers |

outnumber the generations | both before and after them. |
In their youth, | Baby Boomers | caused new schools to open. |
Growing up, | they required more food, | housing, | and consumer goods. |
In their twenties and thirties, | Boomers flooded the labor force. |
Finding more people than ever | vying for the same position, |
they faced big problems | in employment. | In some ways, |
Baby Boomers are better off | than their parents. |
For example, Boomers grew up | with little threat | of diphtheria |
and polio. | One-fourth | are college graduates, | almost twice as many |
as their parents. | Computer literate Boomers | have an edge |
on older workers. | Most Baby Boom women, |
more educated than their mothers, | work outside the home. |
Baby Boomers | tend to be more flexible | and independent. |
They marry later | and have fewer children. |
Baby Boomers have changed society | in many ways, |
and will continue to | for a long time. |

SOUNDS IN CONTEXT: PHRASE BY PHRASE 2

Listen and underline the /p/ sounds. (Note that not all **p** spellings are pronounced /p/.) If the /p/ sound is pronounced with a puff of air, underline it twice.

The postwar Baby Boom has made a very big impact |
on the American population. |
Baby Boomers outnumber the generations | both before and after them. |
In their youth, | Baby Boomers caused new schools to open. |
Growing up, | they required more food, housing, and consumer goods. |
In their twenties and thirties, | Boomers flooded the labor force. |
Finding more people than ever vying for the same position, |
they faced big problems in employment. | In some ways, |
Baby Boomers are better off than their parents. |
For example, Boomers grew up with little threat |
of diphtheria and polio. | One-fourth are college graduates, |
almost twice as many as their parents. | Computer literate Boomers |
have an edge on older workers. | Most Baby Boom women, |
more educated than their mothers, | work outside the home. |
Baby Boomers | tend to be more flexible and independent. |
They marry later and have fewer children. |
Baby Boomers have changed society in many ways, |
and will continue to for a long time.

SOUNDS IN CONTEXT: PHRASE BY PHRASE 3

Listen and underline the /b/ sounds. Then rewind the tape and practice the passage in longer phrases.

The postwar Baby Boom has made a very big impact
on the American population. |
Baby Boomers outnumber the generations both before and after them. |
In their youth, Baby Boomers caused new schools to open. |
Growing up, they required more food, housing, and consumer goods. |
In their twenties and thirties, Boomers flooded the labor force. |
Finding more people than ever vying for the same position,
they faced big problems in employment. | In some ways,
Baby Boomers are better off than their parents. |
For example, Boomers grew up with little threat of
diphtheria and polio. | One-fourth are college graduates,
almost twice as many as their parents. | Computer literate Boomers
have an edge on older workers. | Most Baby Boom women,
more educated than their mothers, work outside the home. |
Baby Boomers tend to be more flexible and independent. |
They marry later and have fewer children. |
Baby Boomers have changed society in many ways,
and will continue to for a long time. |

ON YOUR OWN

Review the **Sound Focus** exercises introduced in this lesson.
Practice **Phrase by Phrase** steps several times.
Record the passage on the next page from beginning to end without stopping.

The postwar Baby Boom has made a very big impact
on the American population.

Baby Boomers outnumber the generations both before and after them.

In their youth, Baby Boomers caused new schools to open.

Growing up, they required more food, housing, and consumer goods.

In their twenties and thirties, Boomers flooded the labor force.

Finding more people than ever vying for the same position,

they faced big problems in employment. In some ways,

Baby Boomers are better off than their parents. For example,

Boomers grew up with little threat of diphtheria and polio.

One-fourth are college graduates, almost twice as many

as their parents.

Computer literate Boomers have an edge on older workers.

Most Baby Boom women, more educated than their mothers,

work outside the home.

Baby Boomers tend to be more flexible and independent.

They marry later and have fewer children.

Baby Boomers have changed society in many ways,

and will continue to for a long time.

Listen to your recording.

Did you stress the correct syllable in each word?
Did you stress the key word in each phrase?
Did you make function words shorter and weaker than content words?
Did you pronounce the sounds /p/ and /b/ clearly?
Did you make a clear difference between /p/ with a puff of air and /p/ without one?
Did you lengthen vowels that come before a voiced consonant?
Did you practice consonant-to-vowel, vowel-to-consonant, vowel-to-vowel linking and consonant-to-consonant holding?
In which of these areas do you need to improve?
In what other areas do you need to improve?

TOPICS FOR ORAL OR WRITTEN COMPOSITION

1. Report on the effect of the Baby Boom on American society in one to three of the following aspects:
   Clothing and fashion
   Consumer goods
   Education
   Employment
   The family
   Financial investment
   Food
   Foreign trade
   Health
   Housing
   Lifestyles
   Leisure and travel
   Work values

2. Describe several ways in which your generation is better off than the previous generation in your country. You may consider the aspects listed in #1 above.

3. Is there a time in the history of your native country when the birth rate increased or decreased rapidly? Describe some of the effects this change had on society.

Chapter 16

The Gift of Sight

VOCABULARY FOCUS

Do you or your classmates know the *italicized* words below? Two of the three words or phrases given afterward are synonyms. One is not a synonym. Cross out the one that is not a synonym. Discuss your choices with a partner.

1. *admonition:*   a. warning   b. criticism   c. praise
2. *apply:*   a. forget   b. make use of   c. employ
3. *contact:*   a. connection   b. distance   c. communication
4. *facet:*   a. aspect   b. side   c. whole
5. *glory in:*   a. enjoy   b. dislike   c. be happy about
6. *hint:*   a. advice   b. suggestion   c. object
7. *means:*   a. method   b. goal   c. way
8. *morsel:*   a. large amount   b. piece   c. bit
9. *orchestra:*   a. symphony   b. solo   c. musical group
10. *perfume:*   a. stink   b. fragrance   c. sweet smell
11. *relish:*   a. joy   b. satisfaction   c. distaste
12. *reveal:*   a. hide   b. make known   c. disclose
13. *strains:*   a. melody   b. photograph   c. tune
14. *stricken:*   a. encouraged   b. hurt   c. injured
15. *tactile:*   a. touching   b. feeling   c. speaking

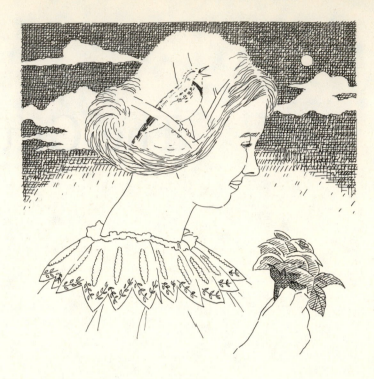

BEFORE YOU LISTEN

Look at the picture and tell what you think.

Describe the objects surrounding the woman.

Which objects in the picture can be known through the sense of smell? the sense of hearing? touch? sight? taste?

Helen Keller (1880–1968) was stricken deaf and blind when she was nineteen months old. Despite her enormous handicap, she learned to understand and use language, eventually graduating with honors from Radcliffe College. She became well-known as an author and lecturer. This passage is an excerpt from her essay, *Three Days to See,* in which she suggests that we live each day *with a gentleness, a vigor, and a keenness of appreciation,* as if we might die tomorrow.[1]

---

[1]Material from *Three Days to See* by Helen Keller is reprinted with kind permission from American Foundation for the Blind, © 1980 by American Foundation for the Blind, 15 West 16th Street, New York, NY 10011.

LISTENING COMPREHENSION

Read these statements. Listen to the passage and choose the best answer for each statement.

1. In this passage, Helen Keller is giving advice mainly to _____.
   a. blind people   b. sighted people   c. deaf people

2. To help us realize that sight is a wonderful gift, we should _____.
   a. imagine we are now blind
   b. use our eyes today as if we would be stricken blind tomorrow
   c. see things even though we are blind

3. Helen Keller admonishes us to touch each object we want to touch as if our tactile sense would _____.
   a. fail   b. fall   c. feel

4. A person can best appreciate Nature's pleasure and beauty by _____.
   a. listening to orchestra music
   b. tasting every bit of food with enjoyment
   c. making the most of sight, touch, smell, hearing, and taste

5. Helen Keller believes that _____ must be the most delightful sense.
   a. sight   b. smell   c. taste

6. Complete the phrases used by Helen Keller by matching the words in the first column with those in the second.

   music _____   a. of a bird
   song _____   b. of food
   strains _____   c. of voices
   morsel _____   d. of an orchestra

LISTENING CLOZE

Listen to the passage again. Fill in the words you hear, one word for each blank. Pause the tape as necessary.

I who am blind can give one (1) _____ to those who see—one (2) _____ to those who would make (3) _____ use of the gift of sight: Use your (4) _____ as if tomorrow you would be stricken blind. And the same (5) _____ can be (6) _____ to the other senses. Hear the music of (7) _____, the song of a bird, the mighty strains of an (8) _____, as if you would be stricken deaf tomorrow. (9) _____ each object you want to touch as (10) _____ tomorrow your tactile sense would fail. Smell the (11) _____ of flowers, taste with relish each (12) _____, as if tomorrow you (13) _____ never smell and taste again. Make (14) _____ most of every sense; glory in all the (15) _____ of pleasure and beauty which the world (16) _____ to you through the several (17) _____ of contact which Nature provides. But of all the (18) _____, I am sure sight must be the most (19) _____.

DISCUSSION

How does Nature reveal pleasure and beauty to us?
Which of your five senses do you use most? Which do you use least?
What is your opinion of Helen Keller's admonition?

SOUND FOCUS 1: /ɑi/

To produce the diphthong[2] /ɑi/, as in *eye,* lower your jaw and tongue as for the sound /ɑ/. As you make a voiced sound, raise your jaw and glide your tongue upward and forward into the sound /i/.

---

[2]A diphthong is made up of two vowel sounds blended together into one syllable.

Underline the letters that make the sound /ɑi/.

I	type	vibrate
eyes	blind	applied
sight	dry	delightful
life	mighty	outside

SOUND FOCUS 2: /ɑu/

To produce the diphthong /ɑu/, as in *out,* lower your jaw and tongue as for the sound /ɑ/. As you make a voiced sound, raise your jaw and glide your tongue upward and backward into the sound /u/.

Underline the letters that make the sound /ɑu/.

out	about	trousers
sound	around	vowel
south	allow	pronounce
crowd	flowers	downtown

SOUND FOCUS 3: /ɔi/

To produce the diphthong /ɔi/, as in *voice,* lower your jaw and lips, and round your lips slightly, as for the sound /ɔ/. As you make a voiced sound, raise your jaw and glide your tongue upward and forward into the sound /i/.

Underline the letters that make the sound /ɔi/.

toy	voices	annoyed
boy	noisy	viewpoint
soil	enjoy	destroy
coin	loyal	rejoin

SOUND FOCUS 4: QUESTION WORD STRESS

When *Wh-* words such as *Who, What, Where, How* are used to ask a question, they are usually placed at the beginning of a sentence and are stressed as a content word. When they are used as relative adjectives and adverbs, they are usually placed in the middle of a sentence and are weaker and lower. Stress the *Wh-* word in the first sentence of each pair. Unstress it in the second sentence.

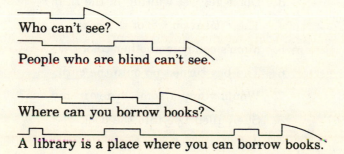

Who can't see?

People who are blind can't see.

Where can you borrow books?

A library is a place where you can borrow books.

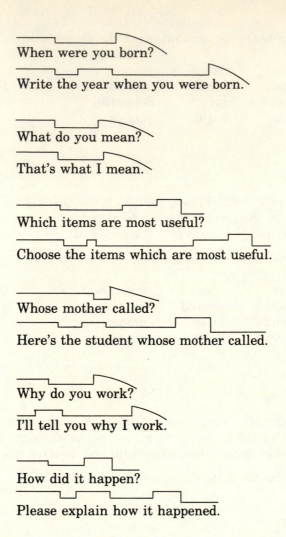

When were you born?

Write the year when you were born.

What do you mean?

That's what I mean.

Which items are most useful?

Choose the items which are most useful.

Whose mother called?

Here's the student whose mother called.

Why do you work?

I'll tell you why I work.

How did it happen?

Please explain how it happened.

SOUND FOCUS 5: VOWEL REVIEW

Practice saying these sentences to a partner. Pay particular attention to the clear and reduced vowel sounds. Stress the content words.

1. Lee sits in this seat.   (/iᵛ/, /ɪ/)

2. Did Lynn say Len was dead?   (/ɪ/, /ɛ/)

3. Don't get wet waiting in the rain.   (/ɛ/, /eʸ/)

4. The cat sat on top of the box.   (/æ/, /a/)

5. Mom's collar is another color.   (/a/, /ʌ/)

6. The bus turned up onto the curb.   (/ʌ/, /ɝ/)

7. Would you put some honey in my cup?   (/ʊ/, /ʌ/)

8. Sue pulled Lou into the pool.   (/uʷ/, /ʊ/)

9. A hawk stood on a hook.   (/ɔ/, /ʊ/)

10.   J<u>oa</u>n b<u>ou</u>ght a b<u>oa</u>t.   (/o^w/, /ɔ/)

11.   D<u>o</u>n g<u>o</u>t up at d<u>a</u>wn.   (/a/, /ɔ/)

12.   S<u>o</u>meone has s<u>u</u>ng the wr<u>o</u>ng s<u>o</u>ng.   (/ʌ/, /ɔ/)

13.   I w<u>a</u>lk to w<u>o</u>rk <u>ea</u>rly.   (/ɔ/, /ɚ/)

14.   The f<u>i</u>rst w<u>o</u>rd is "w<u>oo</u>d".   (/ɚ/, /ʊ/)

15.   The b<u>oy</u> is ab<u>ou</u>t to b<u>uy</u> a t<u>oy</u>.   (/ɔi/, /au/, /ai/)

SOUNDS IN CONTEXT: PHRASE BY PHRASE 1

Listen and underline the stressed syllables in the content words.[3] Then rewind the tape and practice the passage in short phrases. While you speak, clap out the rhythm.

I who am <u>blind</u> | can <u>give</u> <u>one</u> <u>hint</u> | to <u>those</u> who <u>see</u>— |
one admonition | to those who would make full use |
of the gift of sight: | Use your eyes | as if tomorrow |
you would be stricken blind. | And the same method |
can be applied | to the other senses. |
Hear the music of voices, | the song of a bird, |
the mighty strains of an orchestra, | as if you would be stricken deaf |
tomorrow. | Touch each object | you want to touch |
as if tomorrow your tactile sense | would fail. |
Smell the perfume of flowers, | taste with relish each morsel, |
as if tomorrow you could never smell | and taste again. |
Make the most | of every sense; | glory in all the facets |
of pleasure and beauty | which the world reveals to you |
through the several means of contact | which Nature provides. |
But of all the senses, | I am sure | sight | must be the most delightful. |

SOUNDS IN CONTEXT: PHRASE BY PHRASE 2

Listen and mark the places where linking occurs. Then rewind the tape and practice the passage in longer phrases.

I who am blind | can give one hint to those who see— |
one admonition to those who would make full use of the gift of sight: |
Use your eyes | as if tomorrow you would be stricken blind. |
And the same method can be applied to the other senses. |

---

[3]Material from *Three Days to See* by Helen Keller is reprinted with kind permission from American Foundation for the Blind, © 1980 by American Foundation for the Blind, 15 West 16th Street, New York, NY 10011.

Hear the music of voices, the song of a bird, |
the mighty strains of an orchestra, |
as if you would be stricken deaf tomorrow. |
Touch each object you want to touch |
as if tomorrow your tactile sense would fail. |
Smell the perfume of flowers, taste with relish each morsel, |
as if tomorrow you could never smell and taste again. |
Make the most of every sense; |
glory in all the facets of pleasure and beauty |
which the world reveals to you |
through the several means of contact which Nature provides. |
But of all the senses, | I am sure | sight must be the most delightful. |

SOUNDS IN CONTEXT: PHRASE BY PHRASE 3

Listen and underline the /ɑi/, /ɑu/ and /ɔi/ sounds. Then rewind the tape and practice the passage in complete sentences.

I who am blind can give one hint to those who see—one
admonition to those who would make full use of the gift of sight: |
Use your eyes as if tomorrow you would be stricken blind. |
And the same method can be applied to the other senses. |
Hear the music of voices, the song of a bird,
the mighty strains of an orchestra,
as if you would be stricken deaf tomorrow. |
Touch each object you want to touch
as if tomorrow your tactile sense would fail.
Smell the perfume of flowers, taste with relish each morsel,
as if tomorrow you could never smell and taste again. |
Make the most of every sense; |
glory in all the facets of pleasure and beauty
which the world reveals to you through the several means of contact
which Nature provides. |
But of all the senses, I am sure sight must be the most delightful. |

ON YOUR OWN

Review the **Sound Focus** exercises introduced in this lesson.
Practice **Phrase by Phrase** steps several times.
Record the passage from beginning to end without stopping.

I who am blind can give one hint to those who see—

one admonition to those who would make full use of the gift of sight:

Use your eyes as if tomorrow you would be stricken blind.

And the same method can be applied to the other senses.

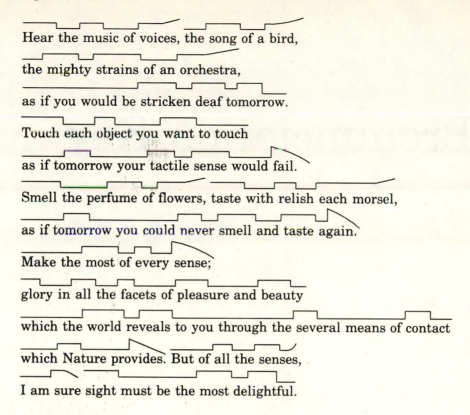

Hear the music of voices, the song of a bird,

the mighty strains of an orchestra,

as if you would be stricken deaf tomorrow.

Touch each object you want to touch

as if tomorrow your tactile sense would fail.

Smell the perfume of flowers, taste with relish each morsel,

as if tomorrow you could never smell and taste again.

Make the most of every sense;

glory in all the facets of pleasure and beauty

which the world reveals to you through the several means of contact

which Nature provides. But of all the senses,

I am sure sight must be the most delightful.

Listen to your recording.

Did you say words together in thought phrases?
Did you make stressed syllables long, strong, high, and clear?
Did you make unstressed syllables short, weak, low and less clear?
Did you pronounce the /ɑi/, /ɑu/ and /ɔi/ sounds clearly?
Did you use good overall stress, intonation, rhythm, and linking?
In which of these areas do you need to improve?
In what other areas do you need to improve?

TOPICS FOR ORAL OR WRITTEN COMPOSITION

1. For ten or fifteen minutes, put yourself at ease in a place where you can concentrate on one or two of your senses (touch, smell, sight, hearing, taste). Choose senses that you do not usually concentrate on. Then describe what you sense.

2. Helen Keller learned to speak, read and write under the guidance of her governess (a teacher who lives in the student's home), Anne Sullivan. Research and tell something about how she succeeded despite her great handicap.

3. Describe how you, or someone you know, overcame a great difficulty in life. Explain the difficulty and how it was resolved.

Pronunciation Key

CONSONANTS		VOWELS	
/b/ baby	/p/ people	/iʸ/ reed	/ʊ/ put
/d/ do	/r/ raft	/ɪ/ river	/uʷ/ shoe
/ð/ this	/s/ side	/eʸ/ say	/ʌ/ cut
/dʒ/ jail	/ʃ/ show	/ɛ/ every	/ɚ/ earn
/f/ fall	/t/ time	/æ/ act	/ə/ away
/g/ get	/tʃ/ chair	/a/ father	/ɑi/ my
/h/ house	/θ/ thin	/ɔ/ ought	/ɑu/ out
/k/ cat	/v/ very	/oʷ/ oak	/ɔi/ voice
/l/ lake	/w/ want		
/m/ sum	/y/ yes		
/n/ sun	/z/ zoo		
/ŋ/ sung	/ʒ/ measure		

NOTE:

A dot over a vowel indicates a syllable: around.

An accent over a vowel indicates a stressed syllable: around.

A slash through a vowel indicates a reduced vowel: around.

A curved line joining sounds in two words indicates linking: have an apple.

A bracket joining sounds in two words indicates holding: last time.

A line above a phrase indicates intonation: She's a student.

Pronouncing Glossary

Each vocabulary word or expression is followed by the pronunciation used in *Phrase by Phrase*. The number indicates the lesson in which it was introduced.

accident	æksidənt	11
accomplish	əkámpliʃ	9
active	æktiv	12
admonition	ædməníʃən	16
adventure	ədvéntʃɚ	10
agreeable	əgriyəbəl	13
ambulance	æmbyʊləns	11
analyze	ænəlɑiz	14
ant	ænt	1
apply	əplái	16
anyway	ɛniwey	13
article	ártikəl	9
ash	æʃ	12
avalanche	ævəlæntʃ	12
avoid	əvɔid	11
be dying to	bidɑiŋtʊ	6
be good at	bigʊdət	3
beautiful	byúʷtifəl	1

benevolent	bənɛ́vələnt	13
bicyclist	báisɨklɪst	11
blanket	blǽŋkət	10
blare	blɛr	11
boom	búʷm	15
bough	báu	7
bow	báu	7
break in	breʸkín	6
breeze	briʸz	7
bruised	brúʷzd	11
bulge	bʌ́ldʒ	15
can't help	kǽnt hɛ́lp	4
cavern	kǽvɚn	10
cereal	sírɪəl	2
chat	tʃǽt	13
cheek	tʃiʸk	8
cheerfully	tʃiʸrfəli	13
chest	tʃɛ́st	2
chop	tʃɑp	3
chopsticks	tʃɑpstɪks	3
chuckle	tʃʌ́kəl	13
cliff	klɪf	10
cloudy	kláudi	1
comfort	kʌ́mfɚt	8
communicate	kəmyúʷnikeʸt	8
complex	kɑmplɛ́ks	9
compound	kɑ́mpɑund	8
computer literate	kəmpyúʷtɚ lítɚit	15
concern	kənsɚ́n	9
concept	kɑ́nsɛpt	14
consist	kənsíst	8
constant	kɑ́nstənt	9
consumer	kənsúʷmɚ	15
consumer goods	kənsúʷmɚ gʊdz	15
contact	kɑ́ntækt	16
converse	kənvɚ́s	8

creative	kriéᵛtiv	14
crops	krɑps	12
daisy	déᵛzi	5
damage	dǽmidʒ	12
daydream	déᵛdriᵛm	11
decade	dέkeᵛd	12
delight	dilɑ́it	4
depression	diprέʃən	15
destruction	distrʌ́kʃən	12
device	divɑ́is	14
diet	dɑ́iət	2
dignified	dígnifɑid	7
diphtheria	difθírìə	15
dive	dɑiv	13
drag	dræg	13
dumpling	dʌ́mpliŋ	3
duty	dúʷti	4
east	iᵛst	6
embrace	imbréᵛs	4
encouragement	inkɚ́idʒmənt	9
end up	ɛndʌ́p	11
enjoy	indʒɔ́i	1
erupt	irʌ́pt	12
excuse	ikskyúʷs	11
exercise	έksɚ̀sɑiz	2
expert	έkspɚt	10
explode	iksplóʷd	12
facet	fǽsit	16
familiar	fəmílyɚ	13
feel like	fiᵛlɑik	3
fertilizer	fɚ̀tilɑizɚ	5
figure out	fígyɚɑut	6
finally	fɑ́inəli	1
firm	fɚ̀m	7
fishing rod	fíʃiŋ	6
flexible	flέksibəl	15

flip	flɪp	10
float	floʷt	10
flood	flʌd	15
fold	foʷld	13
fortunately	fɔ́rtʃənɪtli	12
frisbee	frízbi	6
further	fɚ́ðɚ	4, 9
gaze	geʸz	1
gear	giʸr	6
generation	dʒɛnəréʸʃən	15
genius	dʒíʸnyəs	14
geology	dʒiʸálədʒi	12
get along	gɛtəlɔ́ŋ	6
glare	glɛ́r	11
glory	glɔ́ri	16
gopher	goʷfɚ	13
gorilla	gərílə	8
grasshopper	grǽshapɚ	1
grip	grɪp	13
have an edge on	hǽvənɛ́dʒɔn	15
heart	hɑrt	4
hike	hɑik	6
hint	hɪnt	16
hop	hɑp	11
horn	hɔrn	11
hose	hoʷz	5
howl	hɑul	11
hug	hʌg	8
humble	hʌ́mbəl	7
impact	ímpækt	15
impressed	imprɛ́st	5
independent	indəpɛ́ndənt	15
inspiration	inspəréʸʃən	14
inspire	inspɑ́ir	5
jogging	dʒɑ́gɪŋ	2
juicy	dʒúʷsi	2

kid	kɪd	5
kinetoscope	kɪnɛtəskoʷp	14
kiss	kɪs	8
kitten	kɪtn̩	8
labor force	leʸbɚfɔrs	15
lightning	lɑitnɪŋ	7
look after	lʊkæftɚ	4
make a mark	meʸkəmɑrk	9
master	mæstɚ	4
matter	mætɚ	3
means	miʸnz	16
meanwhile	miʸnwɑil	5
measure	mɛʒɚ	12
mighty	mɑiti	7
model	mɑdəl	9
modest	mɑdist	14
morsel	mɔrsəl	16
Mother Nature	mʌðɚneʸtʃɚ	13
motion picture	moʷʃənpɪktʃɚ	14
mountain range	mɑuntnreʸndʒ	12
mow	moʷ	5
mud	mʌd	12
mushroom	mʌʃruʷm	3
name calling	neʸmkɔlɪŋ	4
napkin	næpkɪn	8
neighbor	neʸbɚ	5
oak	oʷk	7
old fogy	oʷldfoʷgi	13
orchestra	ɔrkəstrə	16
ought to	ɔtə	6
outing	ɑutɪŋ	6
outnumber	ɑutnʌmbɚ	15
pack	pæk	6
patch	pætʃ	5
patent	pætn̩t	14
pay attention	peʸətɛnʃən	1

perfect	pɚ́fɪkt	4
perfume	pɚ̀fyúʷm	16
perspiration	pɚ̀spəréʸʃən	14
phonograph	fóʷnəgræf	14
plant	plǽnt	13
poke	póʷk	13
polio	póʷlioʷ	15
postwar	póʷstwɔr	15
practically	prǽktɪkəli	3
prawn	prɔ́n	3
pride	prɑ́id	7
process	prɑ́sɛs	14
provide	prəvɑ́id	9
publish	pʌ́blɪʃ	9
purpose	pɚ́pəs	9
push-up	púʃʌp	2
question	kwɛ́stʃən	7
raft	rǽft	10
rake	réʸk	5
realize	ríʸəlɑiz	2
recognize	rɛ́kəgnaiz	14
reeds	ríʸdz	7
refrigerator	rɪfrɪ́dʒəreʸtɚ	3
relationship	rɪléʸʃənʃɪp	14
relax	rɪlǽks	2
relish	rɛ́lɪʃ	16
remain	rɪméʸn	4
reply	rɪplɑ́i	1
research	ríʸsɚtʃ	9
restaurant	rɛ́stərɑnt	3
result	rɪzʌ́lt	5
reveal	rɪvíʸl	16
reward	rɪwɔ́rd	9
right	rɑ́it	1
rim	rɪ́m	7
rotate	róʷteʸt	2

rough	rʌf	4
ruin	rúʷɪn	7
satisfaction	sӕtɪsfӕkʃən	9
sausage	sɔsɪdʒ	2
serve	sɚv	9
severe	sɪvíʸr	12
shed	ʃɛd	5
sheepishly	ʃíʸpɪʃli	11
shoulder	ʃóʷldɚ	2
sign language	sáɪnlӕŋgwɪdʒ	8
silent	sáɪlənt	10
sit-up	sítʌp	2
skin	skɪn	3
sneak up	sníʸkʌp	11
society	səsáɪəti	9
soy sauce	sɔɪsɔs	3
sparkle	spárkəl	4
spectacular	spɛktӕkyʊlɚ	10
spring	sprɪŋ	4
starving	stárvɪŋ	1
stoop	stúʷp	7
store	stɔr	1
strains	stréʸnz	16
stretch	strɛtʃ	2
stricken	stríkən	16
stroll	stróʷl	13
stuff	stʌf	3
suffer	sʌfɚ	1
summer	sʌmɚ	1
superior	sʊpíʸriɚ	7
supermarket	súʷpɚmarkɪt	11
support	səpɔrt	9
survive	sɚváiv	10
sway	swéʸ	7
sweat	swɛt	2
swim suit	swímsúʷt	6

tactile	tǽktəl	16
take a liking to	teykəlɑ́ikiŋtʊ	8
talent	tǽlənt	14
talk over	tɔkóʷvɚ	6
terrific	tərífik	6
thick	θɪk	2
threat	θrɛ́t	15
thrilling	θríliŋ	10
throat	θroʷt	4
toast	toʷst	2
topple	tɑ́pəl	7
treat	triʸt	8
tug	tʌg	13
tulip	túʷlɪp	5
tumble	tʌ́mbəl	10
tune	túʷn	11
urge	ɚdʒ	9
vegetable	vɛ́dʒtəbəl	5
vibrate	vɑ́ibreʸt	4
vie	vɑi	15
viewpoint	vyúʷpɔint	9
vocabulary	vəkǽbyʊlɛri	8
volcano	vɔlkéʸnoʷ	12
weed	wiʸd	5
wheat	wiʸt	12
whirl	wɚl	10
whiskers	wískɚz	8
wrap	ræp	3
would rather	wʊdrǽðɚ	3
yeah	yɛ	3
you bet	yúʷbɛt	6
youth	yúʷθ	14
zone	zoʷn	12